Echocardiography in Metabolic Syndrome

Metabolic syndrome (MetS) is a serious health condition that places people at a higher risk for heart disease, diabetes, stroke, and atherosclerosis. Prevalent worldwide, MetS-related induced mortality frequently contributes to the progression of heart failure, which can however be controlled by proper treatment. This book identifies the echocardiographic characteristics that undergo changes in MetS, significantly affecting its course, and contributing to the clinical aggravation of the disease. This linking with echocardiography as a marker of heart failure due to MetS is useful for academics and professionals in cardiology, endocrinology, and internal medicine for effective management.

Key Features

- Provides practical guidance for the management of patients with MetS using echocardiography
- Focuses on innovative methods of prevention and treatment to control the disease using case scenarios, working as a quick reference for cardiologists, electrophysiologists, endocrinologists, and clinicians
- Imparts perspectives of ongoing debates and controversies about the role of echocardiography in the management of MetS

Echocardiography in Metabolic Syndrome
Monitoring and Management

David Maisuradze
and Alexandre Qistauri

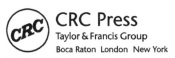

CRC Press
Taylor & Francis Group
Boca Raton London New York

CRC Press is an imprint of the
Taylor & Francis Group, an **informa** business

Cover image Shutterstock ID 1711814788

First edition published 2024
by CRC Press
6000 Broken Sound Parkway NW, Suite 300, Boca Raton, FL 33487–2742

and by CRC Press
4 Park Square, Milton Park, Abingdon, Oxon, OX14 4RN

CRC Press is an imprint of Taylor & Francis Group, LLC

Library of Congress Cataloging-in-Publication Data
[Insert LoC Data here when available]

ISBN: 978-1-032-55948-3 (hbk)
ISBN: 978-1-032-55941-4 (pbk)
ISBN: 978-1-003-43301-9 (ebk)

DOI: 10.1201/9781003433019

Typeset in Sabon LT Pro
by Apex CoVantage, LLC

To my parents
D.M.

Contents

Author Biographies

Dr. David Maisuradze is the leading cardiologist of Aversi Clinic. Aversi Clinic is a medical ambulatory-polyclinic institution in the Republic of Georgia corresponding to world standards, outfitted with the newest medical equipment and technologies. In 2006, he was granted the title of "European Cardiologist." In 2007, he received the title of Fellow of European Society of Cardiology (ESC) and in 2020 Fellow of European Association of Cardiovascular Imaging (EACVI). Dr. Maisuradze completed his doctoral dissertation in 2022. As an active member of American Society of Echocardiography (ASE) and ESC, he has participated in different trials. He has published several articles and clinical cases in various journals.

Professor Alexandre Oistauri is an Emeritus Professor of Tbilisi State Medical University. He is the author of 150 scientific works and 3 books. Over 1993–2014, he provided scientific, practical guidance to the therapeutic clinic of Tbilisi Railway Central Hospital; since 2015, he has been leading the Department of Internal Medicine of the First University Clinic of Tbilisi State Medical University (TSMU). Professor Qistauri is a doctor of medical sciences, professor, and academician. A priority treatment direction for diabetic ankle and diabetic osteoarthropathy has been developed. The topic of the candidate's thesis—"Bone Pathology in Patients with Diabetes" was defended in 1982. The topic of the doctoral thesis—"Pathogenesis and Complex Treatment of Calcium Homeostasis Disorders in Patients with Diabetes" was defended in 1991.

Introduction

Relevance of the Topic

The term "metabolic syndrome" (MetS) refers to a cluster of disorders characterized by central obesity, impaired glucose tolerance, hypertension, and atherogenic dyslipidemia.

MetS is a widespread condition in the adult population that is of increasing interest to clinical medicine specialists, including primary care professionals. The importance of the topic is due to the global epidemic of non-communicable diseases, which are closely related to such components of the MetS as diabetes and obesity and associated cardiovascular diseases (CVDs)—the main cause of mortality and economic burden in the world and in the vast majority of countries separately.

A separate component of MetS (arterial hypertension, dyslipidemia, obesity) accounts for the main share of the most important risk factors calculated by the WHO. The same trend is seen in the mortality structure of the population of Georgia in 2002, which is reflected in the 2005 WHO report (The European Health Report, 2005, Public Health Action for Healthier Children and Populations [World Health Organization, Regional Office for Europe, Copenhagen, Denmark, 2005]). Approximately 20–25% of the world's adult population has MetS (1).

A study of risk factors conducted in 2007 confirmed the wide distribution of the mentioned factors in the adult population of Didube-Chugureti district of Tbilisi, which indicates the need for even more prevention and effective management of MetS in the near future (2).

Improving the knowledge of primary care professionals about risk factors and providing patient education is important for the prevention and effective management of MetS.

MetS-related mortality and the incidence of MetS are increasing worldwide. Epidemiological studies in recent years confirm that MetS can be considered as one of the epidemics of the 21st century.

As of 2019 (3), there were 463 million cases of MetS, type 2 diabetes mellitus (T2DM), and type 1 diabetes mellitus (T1DM) among adults aged 20 to 79 years. Based on these data, the same indicator in 2030 is expected to be 578.5 million and that in 2045, it is expected to be 700.2 million (3). It should be taken into account that the surrounding environment of a person (place of residence or geographical location) affects the emergence and course of this pathology. Along with environmental conditions, work and working conditions, hygiene, and social conditions should be taken into account (3,5).

Insulin resistance (IR) and T2DM lead to various functional, metabolic, and structural changes, which in turn lead to myocardial damage and progression of heart failure (HF) (4).

In particular, changes in contractile proteins and relaxation disorders, cellular damage, microvascular dysfunction, and neurohormonal and sympathetic nervous system activation are the main mechanisms accompanying IR and DM in HF patients (6).

Each component of MetS contributes to the progression of HF. Proper treatment of MetS reduces the possibility of developing HF. Optimal management of MetS in HF patients reduces morbidity and mortality. Management of patients with MetS and HF by a multidisciplinary team is preferred. Future studies are needed to determine better treatment methods in patients with MetS and HF (7).

Echocardiography is the first-line investigation method for studying the structural and functional cardiac changes associated with MetS and T2DM.

Increased left ventricular (LV) mass, diastolic dysfunction, and changes in left atrial deformation have been described in the course of asymptomatic T2DM and are associated with a poor prognosis (96).

Patients with T2DM without CAD are characterized by myocardial fibrosis. Right ventricular (RV) diastolic function indices and Tei index have been reported to have changed during MetS.

Obesity has implications for left ventricle remodeling and function (97).

The closest visualization methods have not yet been implemented in daily practice (4).

As the review of the literature indicates, changes in all indicators of systolic and diastolic function of the left and right ventricles during MetS have not been studied.

At the same time, new parameters have not been fully studied, for example, parameters of tissue Doppler echocardiography, longitudinal strain, indicators of mechanical dispersion, and parameters of diastolic function.

All of the aforementioned parameters determine the relevance of the discussed topic.

Research Goal and Work Tasks

The aim of the study was to reveal the echocardiographic features that undergo changes during MetS, significantly affect the course of MetS, lead to the clinical severity of the disease, increase the frequency of exacerbations; analysis of these echocardiographic features will significantly improve the clinical management of patients with MetS.

In order to achieve this goal, the following tasks were planned:

1. Study of echocardiographic parameters during MetS based on the medical literature published in the past 10 years.
2. Comparison of the results obtained with the results of traditional echocardiography conducted by us.
3. Determination of new echocardiographic parameters of tissue Doppler echocardiography, global longitudinal strain (GLS), and mechanical dispersion indicators and their comparison with the parameters in the literature.
4. According to the analysis of the results obtained, determination of the existing echocardiographic parameters during MetS, using which it is possible to evaluate and monitor the clinical condition developed during MetS.

Scientific News

On the basis of the research conducted, echocardiographic changes during MetS were studied; for the first time, relatively new indicators were investigated in relation to traditional echocardiographic parameters, such as longitudinal systolic parameters of the left ventricle determined by color tissue Dopplerography and deformation index; GLS was determined by speckle-tracking method; the index of mechanical dispersion as a parameter reflecting the heterogeneous contractility of the LV wall segments (54) of MetS was detected. The so-called risk stratification of MetS was detected according to echocardiographic parameters—in particular GLS and the ratio of early and late diastolic velocities of the septal wall of the mitral ring defined by color tissue Doppler echocardiography -*é/á*sept, which, with other parameters such as EF, mitral annulus peak systolic excursion in M-mode (MAPSE), TAPSE, MechD, s's, s 'l, *é/á*lat), can be determined as the predominant indicators reflecting the structural-functional changes of the heart during MetS.

Along with this—in the case of normal values of GLS (–20%)—there was a decrease in the values of separate segments, mainly lower-inferior/septal segments.

The results obtained should significantly contribute to improving the management of the disease and improving the prognosis by affecting modifiable predictors.

Manuscript Structure and Volume

The thesis includes an introduction followed by a discussion of the literature review, characterization of clinical material, research material and methods, results obtained and their discussion, conclusions, practical recommendations; it concludes with a list of the literature used, which includes 153 sources. The text includes 5 tables, 22 images, and 1 diagram.

1 Literature Review

General Section

A sharp increase in MetS and T2DM has been observed in recent decades.

CVD is the most common cause of death globally and a significant contributor to morbidity, accounting for 17.8 million deaths, 330 million life-years lost, and 35.6 million years of disability worldwide (35,36,37). In addition to the burden of mortality and morbidity, CVD causes significant economic costs, with an estimated impact of €210 billion per year in the EU economy (38). MetS refers to a combination of physiological co-occurrences and interrelated risk factors that place an individual at high risk for CVD and T2DM (39,40). The main components of MetS are central obesity, elevated blood pressure, high triglycerides, low levels of high-density lipoprotein (HDL) cholesterol, and glucose intolerance.

The presence of at least three of the aforementioned risk factors is generally accepted to establish a diagnosis of MetS.

In addition to lifestyle factors, obesity is influenced by genetics.

Twin studies and adoption studies have shown that genetic factors have a significant influence on body mass index (41,47) and that parental obesity is a significant risk factor for offspring obesity. Genome-wide association studies have identified nearly 150 genetic variants that are significantly associated with body size or obesity risk (42,43).

Many researchers have described the role of the immune system in metabolic diseases (46).

It is known to be a chronic inflammatory condition characterized by increased serum levels of various pro-inflammatory cytokines (e.g., tumor necrosis factor-alpha [TNF-α] and interleukin 1-β) and biomarkers of inflammation (e.g., C-reactive protein)

DOI: 10.1201/9781003433019-1

(44). Therefore, significant research is being done to identify the causes of MetS as a chronic inflammation.

Three main organs are the initiators of inflammation in MetS: liver, intestines, and fat depot. Factors such as metabolic stress, exposure to chronic caloric excess, and resulting cell death can induce inflammation at each of these sites (46).

The release of inflammatory mediators from one site promotes inflammation in other tissues, thereby exacerbating the chronic inflammatory state and tissue dysfunction/damage (46).

Comprehensive information on inflammatory triggers will help us achieve new diagnostic and therapeutic goals to prevent MetS-related organ damage.

Factors involved in MetS pathogenesis include the following: innate immunity, overproduction of pro-inflammatory cytokines (TNF-α produced in the liver and adipose tissue in MetS), disruption of enteric molecular signaling, and loss of anti-inflammatory defenses (45).

The association of MetS and T2DM with CVD has been established, but there has been renewed interest in MetS and visceral obesity, as it has also been associated with chronic conditions such as brain diseases and some types of cancer (48–51).

The pathophysiologic background of myocardial impairment in metabolic diseases is multifactorial. Metabolic derangements play a central role among a broad spectrum of putative mechanisms responsible for cardiac structural and functional alterations. Predominant changes in cardiomyocyte energetics, with a significant reduction in glucose supply and utilization, are associated with the depletion of the sarcolemmal glucose transporter type 4, with inhibition of pyruvate dehydrogenase by increased β-oxidation of free fatty acids (FFA), and with TNF-α-mediated dysfunction of insulin receptors (7). Direct or indirect effects of hyperglycemia, excess FFA, and triglyceride uptake and accumulation in cardiomyocytes, oxidative stress, and IR have been widely recognized to contribute to myocardial alterations in metabolic diseases.

RV Dysfunction

Patients with T2DM or obesity demonstrate abnormalities of RV systolic and diastolic function, which have been evidenced by tissue Doppler and strain imaging (30,31). These changes are independent of comorbidities (e.g., sleep apnea), although sleep-disordered breathing may potentiate RV dysfunction in obesity through the increase in pulmonary artery pressure in response to hypoxia-induced vasoconstriction of small pulmonary arteries (31). As demonstrated, disturbances of RV performance may correlate with exercise capacity; however, their prevalence has not been established and their clinical significance remains uncertain (60).

Prolactin, cortisol, free thyroxine, and thyrotropin reflect the pathogenic and clinical features of the course of MetS, particularly in the setting of ischemic heart disease and T2DM, which has diagnostic and prognostic value (101).

MetS is characterized by obesity, inflammatory conditions, hypertension, IR, atherosclerotic dyslipidemia, and endothelial dysfunction. These processes are connected by different hormones, cytokines, and adipokines. Leptins, adiponectins, plasminogen activator-inhibitor-1, and TNF also participate in these processes.

A new factor, which was first described in 2016 by S. Romere, is a starvation-induced glycogenic protein hormone-asprosin (asprosin).

Asprosin is associated not only with MetS factors such as glucose and lipid metabolism, IR, obesity, and inflammation but also with diabetic retinopathy, polycystic ovary syndrome, and anorexia nervosa (9).

Although obesity is a well-recognized risk factor for HF, increasing evidence suggests an opposite prognostic impact of obesity on patients with HF. In fact, several investigations reported that an "obesity paradox" exists among patients with HF, wherein those with higher BMI have more favorable survival rates than those with lower BMI, despite higher rates of hypertension and DM (139–142). Oreopoulos et al. (139), in a meta-analysis of 28,209 patients with HF, reported that mortality of overweight and obese patients was, respectively, 16% and 33% lower compared with patients with normal weight. Cardiovascular mortality was also 19% and 40% lower in overweight and obese patients compared with that in non-obese patients. Association between obesity and HF has been consistently observed regardless of age, gender, systolic or diastolic HF, central or peripheral obesity, and chronic or acutely decompensated HF (140–141). The favorable association of obesity and HF is not simply the result of poorer outcomes in patients with severe HF and cardiac cachexia, as patients with high BMI, whether overweight (BMI, 26–30 kg/m^2) or obese (BMI, 30 kg/m^2), show lower mortality rates than patients with normal BMI and those who are underweight (142). Notably, patients who are overweight or obese before development of HF have lower mortality after the onset of HF compared with patients with normal BMI (142). We also recently reported that multiple sclerosis (MS), defined by ADF criteria that mandatorily include obesity, is associated with improved survival in HF patients (143). Interestingly, HF patients with MS but without DM showed the best survival compared with HF patients without DM and MS and with HF patients with DM but without MS, who showed the worst survival. These observations suggest that IR and not overweight unfavorably affects prognosis in HF patients and are consistent with previous observations that have reported that normal weight individuals with MS carry increased risk of developing HF compared with obese individuals without MS (144). The favorable prognostic association between obesity, MS, and HF is not completely understood, and it remains to be definitively assessed whether it reflects a true protective effect, since this distinction would be relevant in the context of therapeutic management. Mechanistic hypotheses explaining improved survival in overweight and obese patients with HF mainly rely on the balance between the anabolic and the catabolic burdens. The cardiac cachexia observed in end-stage HF is associated with an abnormal cytokine and neurohormone profile with increased risk of mortality (145). In fact, in advanced stages of HF, a condition known as malnutrition inflammation complex syndrome (MICS) is commonly observed and represents the link among cardiac cachexia, weight loss, and increased mortality. The main feature of MICS is the activation of multiple inflammatory pathways that lead to wasting syndrome and hypo-albuminemia (146). In cardiac cachexia, an increased production of TNF-α and cytokine activation have been demonstrated with consequent endotoxin absorption or reduced clearance, so that malnourished HF patients are more predisposed to infections, inflammatory activation, and poor outcome (146). Hence, the presence of a condition that counterbalances the effects of inflammation and protein malnutrition, as overweight or moderate obesity, may be beneficial in patients affected by HF. However, it is less clear whether intentional changes of BMI in patients with HF, either weight gain or weight loss, are associated with CV risk modification. In fact, several observations indicate that unintended weight loss (at least 5% of baseline weight) is associated with poorer prognosis in HF patients, likely reflecting wasting conditions (147). In contrast, no conclusive studies are available that adequately investigated the prognostic impact of programmed weight reduction in obese HF patients. Similarly, unwanted weight gain, reflecting deteriorating hemodynamic status, is associated with a worse prognosis in HF patients (148), whereas no studies have assessed the prognostic implication of adipose tissue increase in underweight or normal weight HF patients. Thus, future research is obviously needed in this context. However, the possibility should not be overlooked that the inverse association between obesity or MS and prognosis in HF patients may merely reflect a collider stratification bias, whereby patients with HF and obesity and/or MS represent a selected subset of HF patients in whom other confounder risk factors associated with worse survival in HF are less represented, resulting in a biased favorable association of obesity and MS with HF in analyses not adequately adjusted for confounder risk factors. In addition, earlier symptoms and signs (dyspnoea, edema) fostered by obesity may result in precocious identification of LV dysfunction, with resultant more aggressive treatment and better prognosis (9).

MetS is strongly associated with the development of HF. Visceral adipose tissue is the primary trigger, accompanied by chronic inflammation, IR, and neurohormonal activation. Each component of MetS contributes to the progression of HF. Proper treatment of MetS reduces the chance of developing HF, and optimal management of MetS in HF patients reduces morbidity and mortality.

Management of patients with MetS and HF by a multidisciplinary team is preferred. Future studies are needed to determine better treatment methods in patients with MetS and HF.

Carotid-femoral pulse wave velocity is currently the most widely used index to characterize arterial stiffness in patients with MetS (10).

MetS and thyroid dysfunction are common in clinical practice.

The development of MetS and weight gain, according to separate studies, lead to an increase in TSH. Impaired glucose metabolism may be associated with hyperthyroidism, decreased thyroid function or increased TSH, and an increase in triglycerides. Hypo and hyperthyroidism are related to a/hypertension. The relationship between thyroid and MetS components is complex and not fully understood (11).

MetS causes pulmonary artery dysfunction and exercise-induced pulmonary hypertension due to mitochondrial dysfunction in patients with normal ejection fraction (EF), which can be ameliorated by empagliflozin (12).

Teixeira et al. observed an inverse relationship between the level of lipoprotein a and MetS in CAD patients (13).

Patients with MetS showed increased cardiometabolic parameters and leukocyte activation after 16 weeks of physical exercise. Studying the specific response of leukocytes and the response of plasma proteins can contribute to the optimization of patient-oriented preventive programs (14).

Exercise and a diet rich in ω-3 semi-unsaturated fatty acids (PUFA) are recommended at this time, although there is no therapy that effectively restores the impaired glucose metabolism, changes caused by hypertension, and atherogenic dyslipidemia. PUFA are metabolized by various enzymes into bioactive metabolites with anti- and pro-inflammatory activity.

An important class of PUFA-metabolizing enzymes is the cytochrome P450 enzymes, which can produce a group of bioactive products, most of which have protective/anti-inflammatory and insulin-sensitizing effects in animals (8).

There are epidemiologic data confirming the association between MetS and skin diseases such as the following: psoriasis, acne vulgaris, hidradenitis suppurativa, androgenetic alopecia, acanthosis nigricans, and atopic dermatitis.

The exact mechanism behind the association between MetS and skin disease is unknown, but IR and chronic inflammatory conditions are likely to be involved (15).

Recent studies have demonstrated that MetS and MetS-related components have a significant impact on breast cancer initiation, course, response to treatment, and prognosis. Recent studies have also suggested that low physical activity and a diet high in fat, saturated carbohydrates, and animal protein, leading to the development of MetS, play a critical role in the development of breast cancer (16). Studies indicate a negative impact of MetS on the male reproductive system (17).

MetS requires polypharmacologic treatment, which includes T2DM, hypertension, and dyslipidemia as well as comorbidities. Complex treatments with different medications lead to their interactions and insufficient patient adherence, which can make managing MetS difficult. A multitarget approach reduces the side effects caused by polypragmasia (18).

An EWAS study of allele frequencies showed that four, six, or nine single nucleotide polymorphisms SNPs were significantly associated with the development of T2DM (19).

Subjects with MetS represented patients with a severe course of the disease at the time of infection with COVID-19. In this case, the pathophysiologic mechanism is not completely certain.

The interaction between SARSCoV-2 and angiotensin-converting enzyme-2 facilitates the entry of the virus into the host cell.

The presence of pro-inflammatory cells in patients with MetS contributes to COVID-19-induced immune disturbances, increased inflammation, microvascular dysfunction, and thrombosis.

Obesity was associated with a 2.4-fold increased risk of severe pneumonia compared with normal-weight patients among 383 Chinese patients with COVID-19, after controlling for other risk factors (19).

In the adult population with congenital heart disease, MetS prevails compared to the general population, which contributes to the development of atherosclerotic changes in coronary vessels. Screening of patients with congenital heart disease for MetS is recommended (20).

Population-based and UK Biobank studies have shown that patients with MetS are highly susceptible to SARS-CoV-2 infection.

In the Ecuadorian population, overweight, obesity, and MetS are at 39.5%, 22.3%, and 31.2%, respectively, of the population. An excess of obesity was noted in women; however, in the case of MctS, there was no difference between the sexes. Abdominal obesity and excess HDL cholesterol were detected in women (22).

According to the recommendations of the WHO, impaired glucose tolerance and diabetes are considered risk factors for the development of cardiovascular complications and obesity.

T2DM requires treatment due to its possible regression. In this regard, certain interventions such as diet, lifestyle changes, and drug treatment are considered effective methods.

Bariatric metabolic surgery (BMS) is the most radical way to reduce weight (23). Patients with MetS improve rapidly after bariatric surgery. Improvement of the condition can also be achieved with medication, diet, and physical activity; when non-surgical methods are insufficient, in most cases bariatric surgery can be recommended.

Bariatric surgery effectively targets CV risk factors, but its effect on CVD is not well established. A comprehensive systematic review and meta-analysis of all cohort studies comparing bariatric surgery patients to non-surgical controls evaluated the effect of surgical intervention on CV outcomes (24). This pooled analysis showed that bariatric surgery was associated with a reduction in all-cause mortality (45%) and CV mortality (41%). It remains to be elucidated whether the beneficial action of bariatric surgery is only due to absolute weight reduction or due to additional ancillary effects as well. In this perspective, bariatric surgery is defined "metabolic" to highlight putative mechanisms such as different expressions of gut hormones, enhanced insulin sensitivity, and changes in the gut microbiome that may contribute to its beneficial effects (115).

Randomized, controlled trials are warranted to determine the relationship between MetS, obesity, and bariatric surgery (24).

The risk of atrial fibrillation was significantly higher in patients with MetS, based on a study of 7,830,602 patients enrolled in a study between 2009 and 2016.

A study of 7,565,531 patients with MetS in South Korea identified a relatively high risk factor for the development of atrial fibrillation (25).

Hypertensive patients with MetS had a significantly reduced left atrial reservoir, contractile function, and strain index in the pre-planned ablation period due to paroxysmal atrial fibrillation (26).

Diabetes increases the risk of endogenous TB reactivation and disease activation in infected patients (103).

The study of the molecular mechanisms of T2DM-induced destabilization of the morpho-functional status of the cardiovascular system is a principally relevant scientific-research direction and the driving force for finding new pharmacological targets, which will improve the quality of life of patients with T2DM (102).

Chronic cardio-metabolic assaults during T2DM and obesity induce a progenitor cell imbalance in the circulation, characterized by overproduction and release of pro-inflammatory monocytes and granulocytes from the bone marrow alongside aberrant differentiation and mobilization of pro-vascular progenitor cells that generate downstream progeny for the coordination of blood vessel repair. This imbalance can be detected in the peripheral blood of individuals with established T2DM and severe obesity using multiparametric flow cytometry analyses to discern pro-inflammatory versus pro-angiogenic progenitor cell subsets identified by high aldehyde dehydrogenase activity and a conserved progenitor cell protective function, combined with lineage-restricted cell surface marker analyses. Recent evidence suggests that progenitor cell imbalance can be reversed by treatment with pharmacological agents or surgical interventions that reduce hyperglycemia or excess adiposity. In this state-of-the-art review, we present current strategies to assess the progression of provascular regenerative cell depletion in peripheral blood samples of individuals with T2DM and obesity; we summarize novel clinical data that show that intervention using sodium-glucose co-transporter 2 inhibition or gastric bypass surgery can efficiently restore cell-mediated vascular repair mechanisms associated with profound cardiovascular benefits in recent outcome trials. Collectively, this thesis generates a compelling argument for early intervention using current pharmacological agents to prevent or restore imbalanced circulating progenitor content and maintain vascular regenerative cell trafficking to sites of ischemic damage. This conceptual advancement may lead to the design of novel therapeutic approaches to prevent or reverse the devastating cardiovascular comorbidities currently associated with T2DM and obesity (125).

The link between chronic cardio-metabolic disease and cardiovascular comorbidities and the clinical outcomes of ischemic CVDs, including coronary and peripheral artery disease, myocardial infarction (MI), HF, and stroke, are often considered unavoidable complications that compromise quality of life in patients with T2DM and obesity. CVD was responsible for nearly 18 million global deaths in 2015 (126,127); collectively, CVD remains the leading cause of death worldwide (128,129). It is estimated that 420 million individuals are living with diabetes and 2 billion individuals are considered overweight, 650 million of whom are affected by obesity (BMI >30 kg/m^2). Due to the increased prevalence of T2DM and obesity in an ageing population worldwide, and despite improved pharmacologic and surgical intervention, the incidence of CVD is expected to continue to rise over the next decade (130). The global financial burden of treating diabetes was estimated at $1.31 trillion in 2015 (131), and CVD comorbidities were responsible for nearly one third ($437 billion) of the cost of therapy. Thus, there exists a compelling need to better understand the pathophysiological interrelationship between T2DM, obesity, and the subsequent development of CVD.

As mentioned earlier, subjects affected by MetS are characterized by different metabolic derangements, which may be subclinical at the time of presentation (e.g., impaired fasting glucose) but have the potential to progress to individual clinical entities (e.g., T2DM). As a consequence, correctly diagnosing MetS requires continuous monitoring, since clinical inertia can unfavorably affect both patient compliance to medical therapy and early identification of MetS comorbidities. Furthermore, through time, different diagnostic criteria for MetS have been proposed by medical scientific societies: this ambiguity poses the need for new, unbiased methods based on molecular features. In this context, the metabolome plays a key role, as this set of metabolites is able to vary in a particular metabolic condition such as MetS (hypertension, central obesity, IR, and dyslipidemia), which is dependent on both genetic and acquired factors. The small metabolites generated by this multifaceted metabolic disorder all contribute to the modulation of the metabolome and can be assessed by metabolomics, which in turn allows for the observation of quantitative changes in molecules suggestive of MetS comorbidities. This bio-analytical technique represents a challenge for diagnosing a pathological state and evaluating the prognosis of nutritional therapy on patients suffering from MetS (46). The study of the metabolome could be conducted by both untargeted analyses (e.g., nuclear magnetic resonance [NMR], mass spectroscopy) and targeted analyses such as chromatographic techniques coupled to mass spectrometric detection (HPLC, UHPLC, GC, and supercritical fluid chromatography) (113).

In the diagnosis of MetS, the NMR approach should provide a good alternative to detect an earlier stage of this condition compared to the traditional methods; the latter are useful when the disease status is well established. The biological fluids most commonly used in NMR metabolomic studies are plasma, serum, urine, and feces (116). For human studies, plasma and serum are preferred because they are easy to collect, and their metabolome reflects changes in metabolism at an individual level. Novel promising biomarkers could be metabolites such as glucose, lactate, uric acid, citric acid, p-cresol sulfate, imidazole, histidine, branched-chain amino acids (BCAA), aromatic amino acids, glutamate and glutamine, propionyl carnitine, and lipids. Glucose is a carbohydrate used as a biomarker to diagnose a change in carbohydrate metabolism (glucose homeostasis) involved in IR or T2DM, which is part of the multifactorial nature of MetS. In a recent study, NMR analysis of the urine profile revealed how patients affected by T2DM show metabolome variation in comparison with healthy subjects. This change consists of a decrease in the concentration of creatinine, N-acetyl groups (glycoproteins), allantoin, glutamate and glutamine, and histidine, with an increase in glucose (117). A decrease was observed in other metabolites, such as valine, leucine, and isoleucine (BCAA) as well as N-butyrate, citrate, and lactate, the last-mentioned metabolite being involved in glucose metabolic pathways (118). Thus, lactate represents an eligible marker to diagnose the pathologies characterized by carbohydrate metabolism disruption at an early state of disease. In several NMR studies on biofluids, increased lactate levels have been observed in both the urine and the blood of patients with T2DM, especially in overweight subjects (119). In a metabolomic study that recruited 63 patients with MetS, 82 patients with MetS and asymptomatic hyperuricemia (HUA) without clinical gout (uric acid > 240 µmol/L), and nutrients 2023, 15, 640 9 of 38 61 healthy control subjects; the serum samples were analyzed using H-NMR spectroscopy; the analysis displayed a tendency for metabolic disorders to grow in patients with both MetS along with an increase in serum uric acid. The results showed a significant increase in lipid, TG, and urine glucose levels and remarkably lowered levels of glutamine, trimethylamine, isoleucine, alanine, lysine, 3-hydroxybutyrate, glutamate, citrate, proline, glycine, tyrosine, and 1-methylhistidine (120), a finding that supports a role of uric acid as an upstream inducer in the pathogenesis of hypertension, IR, diabetes, dyslipidemia, and obesity (121). Therefore, it is a useful marker in the diagnosis of the early state of MetS, and it was proposed as one of its diagnostic criteria (122). The disruption in fatty acid metabolism, which usually occurs with MetS, causes an increase of acylcarnitine. Therefore, acylcarnitine could be an NMR-predictive biomarker of T2DM and other pathological pathways involved in the framework of MetS (123). Indeed, the metabolomic analysis conducted on human blood or serum samples allows the qualification and quantification of acylcarnitine, particularly propionylcarnitine (C3), which plays a paramount role in interrupted lipid and amino acid metabolism in patients suffering from MetS.

MetS is associated with a 2-fold increase in risk for CVD, CVD mortality, MI, and stroke and a 1.5-fold increase in risk for all-cause mortality. There is little variation in risk between the NCEP and rNCEP definitions of MetS. There is also little variation in risk for the modified NCEP and rNCEP definitions compared with the original NCEP definition. In addition, our results indicate that patients with MetS but without T2DM are still at high risk for CVD mortality, MI, and stroke. We therefore suggest that MetS does not require T2DM in its definition in order to be closely associated with cardiovascular risk. Our systematic review has identified an important gap in the literature; studies are needed to investigate whether or not the prognostic significance of MetS exceeds the risk associated with the sum of its individual components. We recommend that clinicians use MetS to identify patients who are at particularly high risk for cardiovascular complications. The prevention and reduction of MetS is essential to reduce CVD and to extend life in the adult population (149).

There is a lack of studies that explore the association between dietary habits and MetS. Nonetheless, current evidence has indicated that meal time, meal frequency, skipping meals, and fasting are all associated with MetS. Eating frequent meals and eating in the morning may have a protective effect on MetS. However, eating at night, skipping breakfast, eating one meal per day, and eating irregularly may facilitate the development of risks for MetS in adults. The effects of fasting on the prevalence of MetS are unclear. Understanding the effect of eating habits is as important as understanding the effect of nutrients on health. Further research is needed to understand the association between dietary habits and the development of MetS (151).

The increased incidence of MetS in women at menopause can be mitigated by a healthy lifestyle, including a healthy diet. Nuts are a major component of the Mediterranean diet, which has been selected as a first-choice option for promoting diet-related interventions. There are several species variants in the nut family, but all maintain quite a stable nutrient composition: specifically, unsaturated fat, bioactive (particularly phenolic-related) compounds, and fiber. The benefits associated with each nut constituent relate to general disease mechanisms such as oxidative stress or inflammation and changes in microbiota. A wealth of experimental studies have described the likely protective effects against disturbances in carbohydrate metabolism, lipid profile, blood pressure, and fat accumulation. Confirmation from clinical studies is still a process under development, with often insufficient evidence due to the limited quality of available studies. A beneficial impact on lipids and on carbohydrate metabolism seems a more solid conclusion, and other plausible effects are a potential but minimally reductive effect on blood pressure, together with a likely reduction in the process of fat accumulation and increase in waist circumference associated with menopause (152).

ACEIs and ARBs are recommended for the treatment of hypertension in patients with MetS (110).

Treatment of a/hypertension in MetS is best initiated with a two-drug combination—an ACEI or ARB with calcium antagonists or a thiazide/thiazide-like diuretic. Treatment should be continued according to the appropriate guidelines (111).

For the treatment of hypertriglyceridemia, it is recommended to start treatment with statins in patients at high risk of CVDs. Metformin is considered a first-line drug in the treatment of MetS (113). Metformin in MetS patients is associated with improved diastolic function (114). Long-term administration of ARB improves diastolic function more than Ca channel blockers do (115).

Moxonidine (Physiotensi) effectively reduces blood pressure in combination therapy of AH in patients with MetS (116).

Fenofibrates (Tricor) can also be used in the presence of high triglycerides (112). They prevent macrovascular as well as microvascular complications in patients with MetS. Fenofibrates, as monotherapy or in combination with statins, also prevent the progression of GID and microangiopathy (retinopathy, microalbuminuria). Both as a monotherapy and in combination with statins, fibrates are effective and safe drugs (117).

Originally conceived as diabetes medications, the SGLT2i have shown great promise and continue to deliver on that promise. Just one short year after the EMPERORPreserved trial provided evidence for SGLT2i benefit across the range of LV ejection fraction (LVEF), further unequivocal support for SGLT2i has been delivered by the DELIVER trial (6). Aside from people with HF with preserved ejection fraction (HFpEF), DELIVER studied people with mildly reduced EF (HFmrEF) or improved EF (HFimpEF).

In brief, DELIVER found that at a median of 2.3 years of follow-up, dapagliflozin allocation culminated in an 18% reduction in worsening HF or CV death, with a comparable reduction of incidence of adverse events between the dapagliflozin and placebo groups (132) to <60% or ≥60% (6). By combining the datasets from DAPA-HF and DELIVER, Jhund et al. (7) were able to examine data from over 11,000 participants who had HF with LVEF ranging from 16% to 74%. This pre-specified analysis revealed a 10%–29% relative risk reduction in CV death, all-cause death, major adverse cardiac event (MACE), and total hospitalizations (hospitalization for HF). That the benefits persisted independent of LVEF is clinically meaningful and signals the need to treat symptomatic HF with an SGLT2i unless there are explicit contraindications (132).

Metabolic Syndrome and Echocardiography

After the first report of ultrasound in the diagnosis of CVD by Edler and Hertz in 1954, the use of echocardiography has expanded exponentially over the following decades (92).

The tissue Doppler method is used to determine the velocity of the lateral and medial mitral annulus and the longitudinal movement of the tricuspid annulus.

Currently, the most important clinical data is obtained by longitudinal strain readings through the 2D speckle-tracking method, which is obtained from the apical approach (93,94).

The four variables recommended for the identification of diastolic dysfunction and their abnormal threshold values are the velocity of the mitral annulus e': septal e' <7 cm/s, lateral e' <10 cm/s, mean E/e' ratio > 14, LA volume index > 34 mL/m^2 and peak TR speed > 2.8 m/s (2).

LV diastolic function is normal if more than half of the available variables do not meet the threshold values for identifying abnormal function. LV diastolic dysfunction is noted if more than half of the available parameters meet these threshold values. The result is uncertain if half of the parameters do not meet the threshold values.

When mitral inflow indicators *E/A* ratio and peak E speed are <0.8 and <50 cm/sec, respectively, then the average LAP is normal or low, which corresponds to the corresponding degree of diastolic dysfunction.

LV diastolic dysfunction is usually the result of impaired LV relaxation with reduced or unchanged restorative forces (or early diastolic suction) and increased stiffness of the LV cavity, which increases cardiac filling pressures.

Thus, when conducting an echocardiographic study in patients with potential diastolic dysfunction, a decrease in LV relaxation, a decrease in restorative forces, and diastolic stiffness should be determined. Although not an index of LV diastolic function, abnormal LV longitudinal systolic function can be determined by measuring MAPSE, tissue Doppler-derived mitral annulus systolic velocity, and LV GLS by speckle-tracking.

Several indices of LV and LA systolic and diastolic function have been proposed in recent years, such as LV relaxation and LV and LA filling pressures. In general, patients with HFpEF (HF with normal EF) usually have pathologically decreased LV GLS, so that LVEDP changes directly with LV GLS. A low absolute value of GLS means a greater decrease in the global longitudinal function of the LV (95).

Echocardiography is the first-line research method to study T2DM-associated cardiac structural and functional changes. Left atrial mass increase, diastolic dysfunction, and left atrial deformity changes have been described in the course of asymptomatic DM and are associated with a poor prognosis.

Patients with T2DM without GID are characterized by myocardial fibrosis. Indicators of diastolic function of the right ventricle and Tei index changed during MetS. The closest visualization methods have not yet been implemented in daily practice (4).

The severity of acute MetS was significantly associated with decreased lateral wall velocity $é$. The ratio of early and late diastolic tricuspid flows (E_t/A_t), tricuspid annulus velocity $(E_t/é_t)$, deceleration time (DT), right atrial wall thickness in diastole (EDWT), and epicardial fat thickness were studied in patients with MetS: EFT, Tei index with pulse, and Tissue Doppler (27).

The increased incidence of HF in diabetic patients is more than what can fully be explained by obstructive CAD and traditional risk factors. Damage often occurs at the microvascular level, which then leads to fibrosis and subsequent systolic and diastolic dysfunction. Several studies have demonstrated an independent association between diabetes and LV mass and wall thickness and reduced LV systolic function (112).

GLS is the most robust LV strain parameter, which may now be readily measured using speckle-tracking echocardiography (8). This is more sensitive and specific than conventional 2D EF as a measure of systolic function and can be used to identify subclinical systolic LVD in cardiomyopathies (9). Previous studies have demonstrated that early detection of subclinical LVD by strain imaging is independently associated with long-term adverse outcome in asymptomatic patients with T2DM (10,11). Likewise, diastolic dysfunction and left atrial enlargement (LAE) are potent prognostic markers in HF, although this evidence has focused on HF-free survival. However, the value of screening of asymptomatic T2DM patients for SBHF is undefined; a vital step is to identify the optimal parameters. We hypothesized that in addition to LVH, the presence of impaired GLS, diastolic dysfunction, and LAE predict incident HF in asymptomatic patients with T2DM (113).

According to Ivanovic et al. (28), MetS causes RV diastolic dysfunction; particularly in normotensive patients with MetS, the ratio of transtricuspidal flow velocity (E) to tricuspid annulus lateral wall velocity ($\acute{e}_{lat}$) had decreased.

The presence of diastolic dysfunction of the left ventricle has been indicated by J. B. Lee et al. (29). In particular, in patients with MetS, the excursion of the septal wall of the mitral annulus (E_m) is decreased and the ratio of the transmitted mitral early diastolic flow rate to the average indices of the early diastolic velocity of the mitral annulus ($E/\acute{e}$) is increased.

Tumca Amanda Donohue et al. (30) point out the uninformativeness of the E/A (transmitral flow early diastole/atrial systole) ratio associated with MetS to predict HF.

According to Qin Wang et al. (31), GLS rate has some diagnostic value in determining early myocardial diastolic dysfunction in MetS patients.

According to la Carruba (32), during MetS, there is a development of diastolic dysfunction.

According to J. L. Cavalcanate et al. (29), MetS-associated diastolic dysfunction does not correlate with significant coronary artery disease.

According to Wojciech Kosmala and co-authors, during MetS, echocardiography is the optimal diagnostic method for detecting subclinical changes and monitoring the dynamics of the disease (34).

As the literature indicates, changes in all traditional indicators of the systolic and diastolic function of the left and the right ventricles during MetS are not fully established. As well, such new parameters as tissue Doppler echocardiography, GLS, and indicators of mechanical dispersion have not yet been studied.

Speckle-tracking 2D strain echocardiography is an ultrasound research method; by study of the deformation of the myocardium, it allows for an analysis of the pathophysiological mechanisms of LV dysfunction and early detection of the asymptomatic stage.

Speckle tracking is the fundamental principle of echocardiographic research in various studies observing the movement of spots—acoustic markers formed as a result of natural refraction of ultrasound rays at the boundary of two dense environments. By analyzing this movement in a 2D mode, the movement of the researched segments, the movement frequency (speed), deformation and deformation speed, and the rotational processes of the heart are determined; 2D strain technology provides an opportunity to evaluate the segmental and global contractility of the myocardium as well as its rotational mechanics. This method analyzes the results of the deformation of the myocardium in three planes—longitudinal, circular, and radial—and describes the processes of rotation and twisting/untwisting of the heart.

There is growing evidence that confirms that the study of myocardial deformation by Doppler or speckle-tracking method provides additional information to assess the clinical condition of the subject (65).

Strain and strain rate (SR) are indicators of deformation, which are the main parameters of heart tissue structure and function. These properties can be evaluated using Doppler or the 2D ultrasound technique. Although these measurements are possible in routine clinical echocardiography, their acquisition and analysis still present some technical challenges and difficulties.

Echocardiographic strain and strain velocity imaging have been used to assess resting ventricular function. During ventricular contraction, muscle size decreases in the longitudinal and circular directions (negative tension) and thickens or lengthens in the radial direction (positive tension).

Similar to tissue velocity, strain parameters are most often used to assess myocardial motion from the base to the apex, which is sensitive to mild damage to the subendocardial layer.

Strain rate imaging (SRI) is considered as a valuable physio-logical method to assess myocardial mechanics, in contrast to the tissue Doppler method, which is recommended in the assessment of diastolic dysfunction. Further studies are needed to determine the true value of this exciting and promising method as a routine clinical practice (105).

Tissue Doppler imaging (TDI) has been established as a useful echocardiographic method for quantitative assessment of LV systolic and diastolic function. Recent studies have shown the prognostic role of TDI parameters in major heart diseases such as HF, acute MI, and hypertension. Systolic and early diastolic velocities (E_a or E_m) of the mitral annulus or basal segments (S_m) of the myocardium have been recommended to predict mortality or cardiovascular events. A higher mean S_m value in the basal segments of patients with coronary artery disease is associated with a lower mortality rate.

Echocardiography is the most commonly used non-invasive method for evaluating cardiac anatomy and function. In addition to its commonly established functions, such as confirmation of diagnosis, determination of etiology, screening for complications, and disease monitoring, echocardiography plays an important clinical role in prognostic assessment.

Traditional echocardiographic parameters such as LVEF and restrictive filling pressure have recently been supplemented with TDI.

Peak systolic (S_a) or basal ventricular velocity (S_m) of the mitral annulus reflects ventricular long-axis motion, which is an impor-tant component of LV systolic and diastolic function (4).

Subendocardial fibers play an important role in the function-ing of the long axis, and they are especially sensitive in various diseases and pathologies.

Because the LV apex is stationary, the simple M-method meas-urement of mitral annular peak systolic excursion is a useful and sensitive measure of LV function, which changes rapidly in response to ischemia with LVEF (106).

Deformation imaging, according to some studies, provides unique information about regional and global ventricular systolic function (66). It has been recommended for use to evaluate the mechanical properties of the myocardium in the case of ischemic heart disease, cardiomyopathies, and LV diastolic dysfunction and to detect subclinical myocardial dysfunction in patients undergoing chemotherapy for cancer or valvular heart disease (67).

Strain (*S*) is defined as the deformation of an object compared to its original size. Strain rate (SR) describes the rate of deformation (i.e., how quickly the deformation occurs). Due to its imaging capabilities, the speckle-tracking method shows the dispersion contractions of the myocardium, that is, mechanical dispersion. This new parameter has been proposed as a marker of arrhythmias during various cardiomyopathies (68,69).

In middle-aged patients with T2DM, *E/e* is a superior predictor of MI and stroke compared to HbA1c and GLS and LVEF.

DM is associated with hypertension, coronary artery disease, HF, and cerebrovascular disease. Screening for early signs of atherosclerotic disease allows for timely intervention, which can be beneficial for patients with diabetes.

In 1972, Rubler et al. proposed a definition for diabetic cardiomyopathy, a condition associated with systolic and diastolic LV dysfunction, independent of coronary artery disease and hypertension (71). The study attempted to evidence the common association between diastolic dysfunction and infection with the SARS-CoV-2 virus. This dysfunction can be detected by echocardiography more frequently than expected, even in individuals suffering from postacute and long COVID-19 syndromes, particularly among those with MS and obesity. In most cases, the evolution of diastolic dysfunction is favorable; its echocardiographic parameters evidence significant improvements, in parallel with reductions in the number and severity of persisting symptoms, especially in individuals without MS and obesity. In this category of patients, we diagnosed severe forms of diastolic dysfunction (type 3) more frequently, and they had worse evolutions, with advances made being minimal, suggesting irreversible cardiac damages, such as interstitial fibrosis. This observation suggests that people with increased BMI and MetS should undergo a more comprehensive evaluation, including TTE, in order to potentially diagnose diastolic dysfunction at an earlier stage, when it could be reversible (150).

At this time, the pathophysiological mechanisms that cause ventricular dysfunction are considered to be probably multifactorial.

Increased oxidative stress is a major factor that can lead to microangiopathy, interstitial fibrosis, cellular protein deposition, impaired calcium homeostasis, and the renin-angiotensin system (72–75). Myocardial injury affects diastolic function prior to systolic function. LV systolic function has traditionally been assessed using LVEF for diagnostic and prognostic stratification. However, this method has weaknesses, including dependence on left ventricle loading and geometry, low reproducibility, and low sensitivity for detecting subtle changes in LV function (76–78).

Analysis of Global Longitudinal Strain by 2D Speckle-Tracking Method

GLS of the left ventricle has been shown to be more reproducible. It is more informative than LVEF in predicting cardiac events and all-cause mortality in the general population with and without HF (79–85).

In recent years, technological advances allow study of the strain of individual layers of the myocardium by the 2D-STE method and determination of the longitudinal strain indicators of the epicardium, middle myocardium, and endocardium.

The myocardium is divided into three layers of the myocardium, which consists of circular fibers of the intermediate myocardial layer and longitudinal fibers of the epicardial and endocardial layers. In the early stages of the disease, myocardial damage occurs predominantly in the endocardium. Endocardial stiffness may be a more sensitive measure of myocardial function compared to epicardial or midmyocardial stiffness in various CVDs. However, normal values of stiffness for each layer have not been precisely defined to date (107).

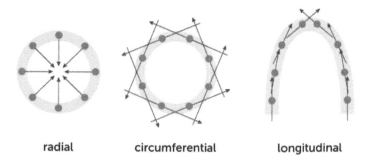

radial   circumferential   longitudinal

Figure 1.1 Heart contraction.

The direction of the LV myofibrils changes from the subendo-cardial right spiral to the subepicardial left spiral.

The geometric shape of the normal left ventricle is considered as a convex ellipsoidal structure with the longitudinal axis directed from the apex to the base.

During the cardiac cycle, the LV wall shortens, thickens, and twists along its longitudinal axis.

Subendocardial myofibrils with a right-handed spiral orientation are shown in purple and subepicardial myofibrils with a left-handed spiral orientation are shown in blue (108).

The torsion of the left ventricle during contraction causes deformation of the matrix of predominantly subendocardial fibers, which leads to the storage of potential energy, which is expended during diastole.

The base and apex of the left ventricle rotate in opposite directions during isovolemic contraction (109).

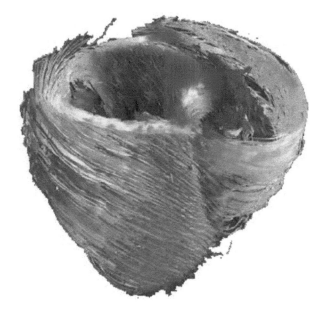

Figure 1.2 Orientation of fibers according to layers.

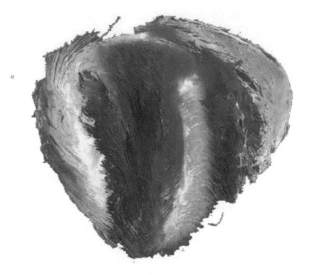

Figure 1.3 Orientation of fibers according to layers.

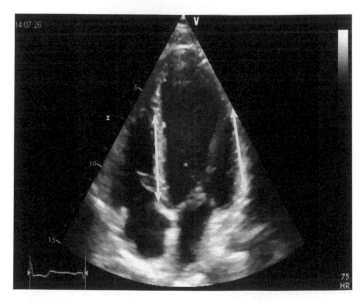

Figure 1.4 Longitudinal contraction of the left ventricule.

2 Characterization of Clinical Material

The work was performed on the basis of the central branch of "Aversis Clinic" LLC and represents the results of the 2017–2020 echocardiographic study of outpatients with MetS.

At the same time, new less-studied echocardiographic parameters of healthy subjects were studied and compared with the same parameters found in the literature and in patients with MetS.

Depending on the goals of the study, both healthy and MetS patients were included in the study at different stages.

The parameters of tissue Doppler echocardiography (50 subjects) and mechanical dispersion (50 subjects) were studied in healthy subjects. The results obtained were compared with the data available in the literature and were included in the control group. At the final stage, 50 patients with MetS underwent a complete echocardiographic study with standard and closest methods.

The results of healthy subjects studied at the previous stages of the research were considered as the control group. Involvement in the study was carried out after anamnestic, clinical-laboratory studies and also after consultation with a therapist, cardiologist, and endocrinologist.

In defining MetS, we were guided by the recommendation of the International Diabetes Federation (3).

Exclusion criteria were as follows: MI, CAD clinical-laboratory and echocardiographic indicators, presence of tumor or pulmonary pathologies in the anamnesis.

DOI: 10.1201/9781003433019-2

3   Research Methods

Standard echocardiography:

- M_modal: 1D ultrasound examination
- B_modal: 2D image of anatomical structures
- Doppler_method: determination of the presence and degree of pathology of the valvular apparatus as well as study of the intracardiac blood flow and pressure ratio
- Color_Doppler_method

Assessment of LV systolic function

- Stroke volume (SV): the volume of blood ejected during one contraction of the heart (measured in milliliters); normally, it is 70–100 mL. Stroke volume is calculated by the formula $SV = EDV - ESV$

  where
  EDV is LV end-diastolic volume
  ESV is LV end-systolic volume

- Minute volume (CO): the volume of blood pumped by the heart in 1 minute (L/min); normally, it is 5–7 L/min. The cardiac output is calculated by the formula: $CO = SV \times HR$

  where
  SV is stroke volume
  HR is heart rate per minute

- Cardiac index: the ratio between cardiac output and body surface area (L/min m^2): $CI = SV/S$
- The surface area of the body is calculated using a special table comparing height and weight: Estimation of Surface Area

DOI: 10.1201/9781003433019-3

from Height and Weight (1991 Scientific American, Anc.) or by Du Bois formula, S = MT 0.423 × P0.725 × 0.007184

where
MMT is body mass (kg)
P is body height (cm)
0.007184 is the constant empirical index

- Stroke volume index: ratio between stroke volume and body surface area (L/min m^2): ISV = SV/S
- M-mode:

  Calculation of LV mass (LV$_{mass}$ – LV mass); MP mass (c) is calculated according to the Penn-convention with the Devereux formula:

  $$LV_{mass} = 1.04 \ [(STd + PWTd + LVIDd)3] - 13.6$$

  where
  STd is the thickness of the interventricular septum in diastole
  PWTd is the thickness of the LV posterior wall in diastole
  LVIDd is the LV diastolic diameter
  LV mass is about 99 g for women and about 135 g for men
  LV mass index (g/m^2): ratio of MP mass to body surface area

- With LV hypertrophy, among the following three criteria—LV mass >198 g, LV mass/height >121 g/m, and LV mass index >120g/m^2—at least two are elevated:

  Relative LV posterior wall thickness (RWT) = 2 × PWT/LVID

  where
  RWT is the posterior wall thickness of the LV
  LVID is the end-diastolic size of the LV

  Based on the parameters mentioned, LV remodeling types are distinguished as follows.

  - Concentric hypertrophy: when LV$_{mass}$ indicators are increased and LV posterior wall relative thickness is $3$0.45 (type I)
  - Eccentric hypertrophy: when LV$_{mass}$ indicators are increased and LV posterior wall relative thickness is <0.45 (type II)
  - LV concentric remodeling: when MP mass indicators are within normal limits and MP posterior wall relative thickness is >0.45 (type III)

- MP geometry is normal when MP mass indicators are within normal limits and MP posterior wall relative thickness is <0.45 (type IV).

- MP final diastolic volume (cm^3): calculated according to the L. Teichholtz formula: $V = [7/(2,4 + D)]D3$

  where
  D is the diameter of the MP cavity (cm)

- Myocardial fiber shortening fraction (FS) is calculated by the following formula:

  FS = (EDD – ESD)/EDD
  %FS=FS × 100%

  where
  FS is the fraction of myocardial fiber shortening
  %FS is the percentage of the shortening fraction
  EDD is the end-diastolic diameter
  ESD is the end-systolic diameter. Normally, %FS is ≥30%

- Evaluation of other systolic parameters of the left ventricle:

  In the M mode, the EF and percent EF (%EF) are calculated using the following formulas: EF = (EDV – ESV)/EDV
  %EF = EF × 100%
  Normally, the EF calculated by this formula is 60–65%.

- B_mode:

  EF and EF percentage were calculated using Simpson's formula to calculate volumes in the apical four-chamber or two-chamber position. This value, calculated by Simpson's formula, is normally >50%.

- Velocity of circumferential fiber shortening (VCF): VCF = FS/LVET

  where
  FS is the fraction of myocardial fiber shortening
  LVET is the firing time
  This indicator can be calculated both in the MM_mode and in the B_mode. VCF is normally ≥1.1.

- Doppler echocardiography method:
- Calculation of stroke volume (SV): SV= CSA × VTI

  CSA = p$d2$/4
  VTI = vcp × ET

where
d is the diameter of the LV outflow tract
vcp is the mean flow rate of the outflow tract
ET ki is the ejection time

Assessment of LV diastolic function:
• Variants of the LV diastolic dysfunction:

  • Delayed relaxation filling pattern (Grade 1): A delayed relaxation filling pattern is commonly seen after the age of 60 years. 13 This filling pattern is characterized by prolongation of the E-wave DT (>200 msec), a reflection of slow and prolonged LV pressure decay that achieves only a modest decline in LV_{min}. As a result, the gradient between the left atrium and the left ventricle narrows, reflected by a low peak E-wave velocity. The small transmitral gradient associated with delayed relaxation limits early diastolic filling, resulting in a residuum in the atrium, which is subsequently ejected into the left ventricle during atrial systole. This increases peak A-wave velocity, a measure of LA stroke volume. The combined effects of a decreased E wave and an increased A wave usually result in reversal of the normal *E/A* ratio, such that $E < A$.
  • Pseudo-normal filling pattern (Grade 2): Progression from type 1b to type 2 filling (pseudo-normalization) is characterized by a rise in mean LAP and largely represents the effects of a further reduction in LV compliance. In contrast to type 1b filling, in which $LV_{operational}$ compliance does not decrease until late diastole, the decrease in operational compliance in type 2 filling occurs in early diastole (at lower LV volume).

• The reduction in early diastolic LV filling seen with grade 2 filling results in an atrial residuum, which increases LAP. This causes an increase in peak mitral E-wave velocity. A concomitant increase in LVEDP produces shortening of A_{dur}. Finally, the increased load imposed on the left atrium as a result of a poorly compliant left ventricle may, over time, lead to decreased atrial contractile reserve, LA enlargement, and a decrease in peak A-wave velocity (reduced LA stroke volume). The combined effects of a rise in *E*-wave velocity and a decrease in *A*-wave velocity result in an *E/A* ratio that is usually >1 (pseudo-normalization).
• Restrictive filling pattern (Grade 3): The transition from pseudo-normal to restrictive filling is characterized by a further decrease in LV compliance, an additional increase in mean

LAP, and the intercession of atrial failure. Worsening compliance causes additional shortening of mitral E-wave DT (to 1.2 m/sec) may fail to demonstrate DT shortening, because of the increased time required for a higher E velocity to decelerate. A continued rise in LAP further increases the peak E-wave velocity, and increased LVEDP is reflected by a short A_{dur}. The increased load imposed on the left atrium eventually results in atrial systolic failure, further LA enlargement, and decreased mitral A-wave velocity. The combined effects of the foregoing E- and A-wave changes further increase the E/A ratio (153).

- LV pressure increases at the beginning of systole. LV chamber stiffness_KV = dP/dV. Normal 0.01–0.025 LV isovolumetric relaxation time (IVRT), which is normally 65 ± 20 msec, although it depends on age:

  <30 years: 72 ± 12 msec, prolongation >92 msec
  30–50 years: 80 ± 12 msec, prolongation >100 msec
  >50 years: 84 ± 12 msec, extension >105 msec

- Prolongation of IVRT indicates prolongation of LV isovolemic relaxation. However, a normal IVRT does not indicate prolonged ventricular isovolemic relaxation, as increased left intra-atrial pressure causes premature opening of the mitral leaflets.
- IVCT isovolumetric contraction time of the left ventricle, which is normally 65–90 msec
- Transmitral diastolic flow, which is normally represented by E/A peaks. Following are the data of different authors: VE = 70–100 cm/c, VA = 45–70 cm/c, E/A = 1.0–1.5, DTE = 160–220 mc
- Half of E peak acceleration time ($AT_{1/2}$), which is normally 62 ± 18 m/c
- Half of E peak $DT_{1/2}$, which is normally 73 ± 24 m/c
- Normal E/A = 1.0–1.5. However, it also depends on age.

- TAPSE

  TAPSE is a measure of longitudinal systolic excursion of the tricuspid annulus. In recent years, tissue Doppler parameters (S wave) and deformation indicators have been distinguished by their reproducibility and are suitable for clinical use, especially for detecting subtle changes and studying systolic function disorders in the preclinical stage of the disease. However, metrics may vary between vendors and software versions (99).

Tissue Doppler is used to determine the rate of longitudinal movement of the mitral and tricuspid annulus.

- Recommended parameters are as follows: s—ventricular systole, e—early diastole, and a—atrial systole.
- 3D imaging systems are becoming widely available.
- Transthoracic imaging used in the assessment of LV size and systolic function.
- EF calculation is the most common 3D software in use today.
- Echocardiographic parameters recommended for the assessment of cardiotoxicity in cancer treatment are as follows:

3D-based LVEF (Figure 3.1)
2D Simpson's LVEF
GLS by STE

Methods of Statistical Analysis

The data wereprocessed statistically using Microsoft Excel 2007. We calculated the average and standard deviation of quantitative indicators. We determined the difference between the indicators using the Student's *t*-test ($p < 0.05$ was considered reliable).

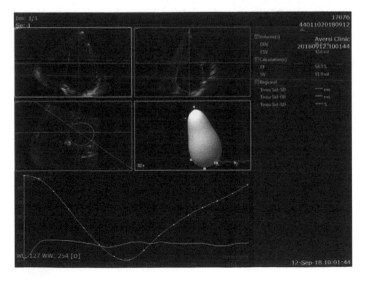

Figure 3.1 3D calculated EF.

4   Results of Our Research

The results obtained were compared with the current guidelines (ASE, American Society of Echocardiography; EACVI, European Society of Cardiovascular Imaging) as well as with the resultspublished in the medical literature over the past 10 years.

Similar to the data available in the literature, our analysis statistically reliably reveals a direct relationship between the pathophysiologic changes developed during MetS and echocardiographic parameters.

Reference values of LV mechanical dispersion assessed by 2D longitudinal speckle-tracking strain in normal subjects

Background

LV mechanical dispersion measured by 2D speckle-tracking echocardiography (MD) is a novel-strain-derived parameter that reflects temporal cardiac contraction heterogeneity and has consequently gained attention as a predictor of increased arrhythmic risk in selected cardiac diseases (55).

LV mechanical dispersion along with LV GLS may provide additional valuable risk markers of VA and SCD in predialysis and dialysis patients (56). LV mechanical dispersion (MD) measured with speckle-tracking echocardiography (STE) is a marker of fibrosis and slow conduction (5).

Our study demonstrated that LV dyssynergy and LV dispersion were strongly associated with the development of fatal ventricular arrhythmias in patients with LVEF ≥35%. In addition, combined

DOI: 10.1201/9781003433019-4

assessment of LV dyssynergy and dispersion can enhance the predictive capability for fatal ventricular arrhythmias in such patients (6).

Mechanical dispersion at 6 months was a strong predictor of ventricular arrhythmias. CRT response by reverse remodeling was dependent on improvement of both longitudinal and circumferential function (7).

LV mechanical dispersion was increased in patients with AS. Increased mechanical dispersion was independently associated with mortality and could confer additional risk (8).

There is increasing interest in assessment of LV mechanical dispersion but normal data are limited (57,4).

Methods

We prospectively studied 50 adult outpatients with normal diastolic function and normal LVEF. A complete 2D echocardiography examination was performed, including speckle tracking with measurements of LV systolic GLS and mechanical dispersion on a commercially available system Epiq7. p value was set significant at <0.05.

Results

- The values of GLS among the studies varied from /–16.7/ to /–24.2%/ (mean GLS = –19 ± 1.59%), p 0.0001 (T.N1)
- The values of MD varied from 1.4 to 33.6 (mean MD: 14.4 ± 8.5), p 0.0002 (Figure 1.1)
- The values of EF varied from 55% to 63% (mean EF: 58 ± 2.5), p 0.0004
- Age of patients varied from 16 to 52 (mean age: 60.8), n = 52, 26% were male, n = 48, 24% were female.

Conclusion

- This study determined values of mechanical dispersion in subjects with a normal EF and normal GLS.
- Further studies are needed to clarify the relation between mechanical dispersion and different cardiac disease.

Reference values of septal-lateral early and late tissue Doppler velocities ratio in subjects with normal diastolic function

Table 4.1 Mechanical Dispersion Data (*N* = 50) in Normal Subjects

Factor	Mean ± SD	p value
Age	60.8 ± 14	0.25
GLS	−19 ± 1.59	<0.0001
MD	14.4 ± 8.5	<0.00001
EF	58 ± 2.5	0.008

Note: p value significant at <0.05.
Abbreviations: SD, standard deviation, EF, ejection fraction.

Introduction

Echocardiography is now the most commonly used noninvasive tool for the assessment of cardiac anatomy and function. In addition to commonly established roles such as confirming the diagnosis, etiologic work-up, complication screening, and disease monitoring, echocardiography plays an important clinical role in prognostic assessment. Conventional echocardiographic predictors of poor outcome, such as LV EF and restrictive filling pattern, have recently been supplemented by TDI. TDI, an advanced echocardiographic modality, is a robust and reproducible echocardiographic tool that has permitted a quantitative assessment of both global and regional function and timing of myocardial events .

Tissue Doppler echocardiography (TDE) is used in the assessment of diastolic function; however, it is unclear whether the medial ($\acute{E}_{med}$) or lateral ($\acute{E}_{lat}$) annulus should be used.

There have been limited studies on the use of TDE in subjects with normal systolic function.

Systolic TDI parameters are complementary tools in the evaluation of LV systolic function, especially in patients with subtle systolic dysfunction despite preserved LVEF.

TDI echocardiography is already a part of the standardized diastolic evaluation. Its ability to detect early signs of cardiac disease before it is detectable by conventional echocardiography and its strong predictive power are encouraging. The late diastolic velocity, *á*, reflects the ventricles' passive motion, which is dependent on the viscoelastic properties.

Echocardiographic assessment of LV diastolic function is an integral part of the routine evaluation of patients presenting with symptoms of dyspnea or HF.

Differentiation between normal and abnormal diastolic functions is complicated by overlap between Doppler indices values in healthy individuals and those with diastolic dysfunction. The four recommended variables and their abnormal-cutoff values are as follows:

- Annular $é_{velocity}$ (septal $é$< 7 cm/sec, lateral $é$ < 10 cm/sec)
- Average $E/é$ ratio > 14
- LA maximum volume index > 34 mL/m^2
- Peak TR velocity > 2.8 m/sec

LV diastolic dysfunction is present if more than half of the available parameters meet these cutoff values. The diagnosis is inconclusive if half of the parameters do not meet the cutoff values. Diastolic dysfunction is a significant predictor of MACEs in the general population. A number of echocardiographic parameters have been shown to reflect diastolic dysfunction. How to interpret these parameters has been widely discussed and numerous classification algorithms have been proposed. However, these algorithms often leave a substantial amount of patients as indeterminate due to incongruent echocardiographic parameters.

Background

TDI detects early signs of LV dysfunction. Diastolic dysfunction also is an early sign of the heart disease. The aim of this study was to define the range of the ratio between the LV septal and lateral early *é* and late *á* TDI velocities in subjects with normal diastolic function.

Methods

We prospectively studied 50 adult outpatients with normal diastolic function and normal LVEF. We used 2D echo, including septal and lateral tissue Doppler *é/á* ratio. We analyzed diastolic function by standard echocardiography, according to the ASE/ EACVI 2016 guidelines together with clinical parameters. An E/A ratio ≤ 0.8 with a peak E-wave velocity ≤ 50 cm/sec indicated grade I diastolic dysfunction.

Results

The values of septal *é/á* among the studies varied from 0.9 to 2.4 (mean 1.33).

- The values of lateral *é/á* among the studies varied from 1 to 2.0 (mean, 1.75).
- The values of E/A ratio varied from 1 to 2.1 (mean, 1.38) (Figure 1.1).
- Age of patients varied from 17 to 51 (mean age, 31); $n = 50\%$, 25 were male; $n = 50\%$, 25 were female.

Conclusion

- We found that septal and lateral mean *é/á* ratio >1 in subjects with normal diastolic function.
- Tissue Doppler *é/á* ratios in patients with diastolic dysfunction require further investigation.
- This study determined septal-lateral tissue Doppler *é/á* ratios in subjects with a normal heart function.

Table 4.2 *é/á* Septal and *é/á* Lateral

Factor	Mean ± SD	p value
Age	31 ± 8.3	0.011
E/A velocity ratio	1.38 ± 0.26	<0.00001
é/á septal	1.33 ± 0.31	<0.00001
é/á lateral	1.75 ± 0.53	<0.00001

Notes: Data ($N = 50$) in subjects with normal diastolic function. p value is significant at <0.05.
Abbreviation: SD, standard deviation.

Does the LV medial tissue Doppler *é/á* ratio add diagnostic value in left ventricle diastolic dysfunction?

Background

Diastolic dysfunction is an early sign of the heart disease. Detection of diastolic disturbances has been predicted to lead to early recognition of underlying heart disease. TDI parameters have shown to be a sensitive marker to detect progressive deterioration of cardiac function in various cardiac conditions. The aim of this research was to calculate the *é/á* ratio of medial annulus in patients with mild diastolic dysfunction and determine their diagnostic value.

Methods

We prospectively studied 50 adult outpatients with normal diastolic function (group I, the control group) and 50 adult outpatients with grade I LV diastolic dysfunction (2016 ASE/EACVI guidelines) and normal LVEF (group II). We determined diastolic function as grade I using four criteria:

- Average E/é > 14
- Septal $é_{velocity}$ < 7 sm/sec or lateral $é_{velocity}$ 10 sm/sec
- TR velocity > 2.8 m/sec
- LA volume or index > 34 mL/m²) or $E/A \leq 0.8 + E \leq 50$ sm/sec

We used 2D echo, including septal-lateral tissue Doppler *é/á* ratio. Standard TTE examinations were performed on a commercially available system Epiq7.

To assess LV diastolic function, the transmitral early (E) and late (A) wave velocities were measured by pulsed Doppler ultrasound at the mitral leaflet tips. Peak systolic (*ś*) and early (*é*) and late (*á*) diastolic velocities of the medial mitral annulus were measured by pulsed tissue Doppler imaging from the apical four-chamber view. The ratio *é/á* was calculated. Data were expressed as mean ± standard deviation. $p < 0.05$ was set as statistically significant.

Results

- Group I: The septal *é/á* ratio among the studies varied from 0.9 to 2.4 (mean 1.33 ± 0.31), $p < 0.00001$ (Figure 1.1).

  - Lateral *é/á* ratios among the studies varied from 1 to 2.0 (mean, 1.75 ± 0.53), $p < 0.00001$.
  - *E/A* ratios varied from 1 to 2.1 (mean *E/A*, 1.38 ± 0.26), $p < 0.00001$.
  - Age of patients varied from 17 to 51 (mean age, 31); $n = 50\%$, 25 were male; $n = 50\%$, 25 were female (Figure 1.2).

- Group II: Septal *é/á* ratios among the studies varied from 0.4 to 0.9 (mean, 0.61 ± 0.12), $p < 0.00001$ (Figure 1.3).

  - Mean LVEF was 56 ± 3% (range 50–61%), p 0.008.
  - The *E/A* ratios varied 0.4 to 0.9 (mean, 0.61 ± 0.12) (Figure 1.4). Age of patients varied from 25 to 91 (mean age, 59.6 ± 14).

Conclusion

- In patients with mild diastolic function, early (*é*) and late diastolic (*á*) pulsed DTI medial velocity ratios decreased compared with those of subjects with normal diastolic function.
- *É/á*$_{med}$: The ratio has good correlation with the *E/A* ratio in patients with mild diastolic dysfunction.
- Future studies are need to determine if the *é/á*$_{med}$ ratio is a useful parameter to evaluate diastolic function.

Table 4.3 Ratios of Early and Late Tissue Velocities of the LV Septal Wall in Patients with Mild Diastolic Dysfunction ($N = 50$)

Factor	Mean ± SD	p value
Age	59.6 ± 14	0.25
E/A	0.71 ± 0.13	<0.00001
É/Á	0.61 ± 0.12	<0.00001
EF	56.4 ± 2.7	0.008

Note: p important < 0.05.
Abbreviations: EF, ejection fraction, SD, standard deviation.

GLS in patients with metabolic syndrome and normal EF

MetS refers to a cluster of disorders characterized by central obesity, impaired glucose tolerance, hypertension, and atherogenic dyslipidemia. MetS is a widespread condition in the adult population that is of growing interest to clinicians, including primary care professionals. The topic is relevant to the global epidemic of non-communicable diseases, which is closely related to components of MetS, such as diabetes and obesity and their associated CVDs—the leading cause of mortality and economic burden in the world and in most countries. Each component of MetS contributes to the progression of HF. Proper treatment of MetS reduces the chance of developing HF. Optimal management of MetS in patients with HF reduces morbidity and mortality. It is advisable to manage MetS and patients with HF with a multidisciplinary team. Future studies are needed to determine better treatment options for patients with MetS and HF. IR and T2DM cause various functional, metabolic, and structural changes, which in turn lead to myocardial damage and progression of HF. Echocardiography is a first-line study method to study the structural and functional changes of the heart associated with MetS and T2DM. As a review of the published literature indicates, changes in all indicators of systolic and diastolic function of the left and right ventricles during MetS have not been studied. At the same time, new parameters such as tissue Dopplerography parameters, longitudinal strain, mechanical dispersion indices, and diastolic function parameters have not been thoroughly studied. The fundamental principle of speckle-tracking echocardiographic examination is the observation of the motion of spots—acoustic markers formed by the natural refraction of ultrasound rays at the boundary of two media of different densities. Speckle-tracking 2D strain echocardiography, an ultrasound examination method, and the study of myocardial deformity can explain the pathophysiological mechanisms of LV dysfunction and the early detection of asymptomatic stage. The GLS analysis using the 2D speckle-tracking method has been shown to be more reproducible and at the same time more informative than LVEF in predicting cardiac events and estimating all-cause mortality in the general population with or without HF . There is growing evidence that the study of myocardial deformity by tissue Doppler or speckle tracking provides additional information to assess clinical condition. Currently, the most important clinical data are obtained by longitudinal strain indices using the 2D speckle-tracking method, which is obtained from the apical approach. Definition of GLS by speckle-tracking echocardiography and longitudinal strain rates in patients with MetS have not been established.

Methods

On an outpatient basis, we studied 50 adult patients with MetS and normal LVEF. Patients underwent 2D echocardiography, including speckle tracking using a measurement of LV GLS. The standard TTE test was performed on a commercially available Epiq7 system. The study included 50 patients with MetS who met the diagnostic criteria for MetS of the International Diabetes Federation (IDF). The online Qlab software analysis was used to analyze each group, including GLS. Exclusion criteria were history of MI, the presence of a history of tumors, or pulmonary pathologies.

Methods of Statistical Analysis

The material was statistically processed using Microsoft Excel 2007. We considered the mean and standard deviation of the quantitative indicators from the mean. The difference between the values was determined by the Student's t-test ($p < 0.05$).

Results

This study evaluated the GLS in individuals with MetS and normal EF. The results obtained were compared with the GLS normal rate (–20%). (6) GLS values in the studies varied from –11.7 to –23% (mean GLS, 16.8%). EF values ranged from 54% to 65% (mean EF, 57.5%). The age of patients varied from 21 to 88 years (mean age, 60.8; n = 19%, 9 men; n = 81%, 39 women). Patients with normal GLS (–18%/–25%) were at 14.29%. Normal GLS (n = 14) segmental longitudinal stretching (LS) between patients was reduced in all patients, from –3% to –14%. Segmental longitudinal strain (LS) decreased in 12 patients in the infero-lateral and in 2 patients in the infero-septal segments.

Conclusion

- MetS has an effect on the functional state of the heart.
- MetS causes a decrease in the average GLS.
- During MetS, in the case of normal GLS, a decrease in regional longitudinal tension is observed.
- STE (speckle-tracking echocardiography) can be used as a reliable method for early detection of LV myocardial injury in patients with MetS.
- Further studies are needed to develop specific therapies that may be more effective in preventing and treating MetS-induced heart changes.

GLS in patients with mild diastolic dysfunction and normal EF

Speckle-tracking echocardiography has proven its superiority over traditional LV markers. Longitudinal strain rates in patients with diastolic dysfunction have not been established.

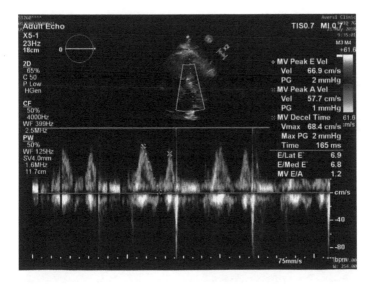

Figure 4.1 Determination of transmitral *E/A* ratio by pulsed Dopplerography.

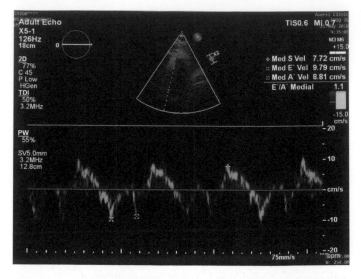

Figure 4.2 Determination of the septal *é/á* ratio by color tissue Dopplerography.

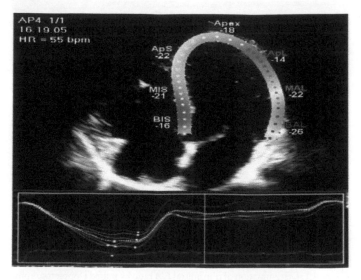

Figure 4.3 Global longitudinal strain (GLS) of the left ventricle.

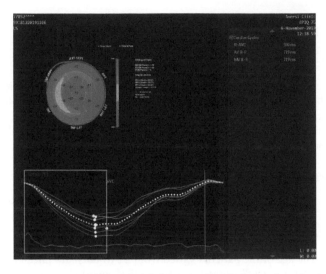

Figure 4.4 Determination of global longitudinal index and mechanical dispersion by speckle-tracking method.

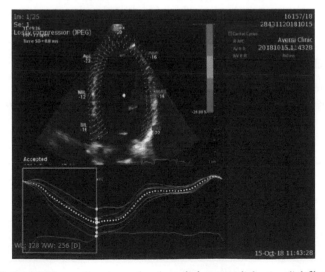

Figure 4.5 Vector directions of endocardial-myocardial-epicardial fibers of the left ventricle during systole.

This study evaluated the longitudinal strain of the left ventricle in individuals with mild diastolic dysfunction and normal EF.

Methods

We studied 48 adults (outpatients) with diastolic dysfunction (class I) and normal LVEF. We performed 2D echocardiography, including a speckle-tracking study measuring LV systolic GLS, as well as a standard TTE examination on a commercially available Epiq7 system.

Results

- GLS values in the studies varied from −11.9% to 211.6% (mean GLS, 16.3%).
- E/A ratios varied from 0.5 to 0.9 (average, 0.69).
- EF values varied from 54% to 65% (average, 57.5%).
- The age of the patients varied from 21 to 88 years (mean age, 60.8; n = 19.%, 9 men; n = 81%, 39 women).
- Patients with normal GLS (−18%/−25%) were at n = 14, 29%.

Among patients with normal GLS (n = 14), segmental LS decreased in all patients, from −3% to −14%. In 12 patients, segmental LS was reduced in the infero-lateral and in 2 patients in the inferoseptal segments (Table 4.4).

Echocardiographic parameters of MetS

MetS and T2DM are prognostic predictors of coronary heart disease (CHD) and mortality (63,65). MetS is associated with

Table 4.4 N4 Values of GLS in Patients with Mild Diastolic Dysfunction (N = 48)

Factor	Mean ± SD	p value
Age	60.8 ± 13.2	NS
E/A	0.69 ± 0.13	<0.00001
GLS	−16.3 ± 2.8	<0.00001
EF	57.5 ± 2.5	<0.00014

Note: p significant <0.05.
Abbreviations: EF, ejection fraction; GLS, global longitutudinal strain; NS, not significant; SD, standard deviation.

increased cardiovascular mortality. But data on cardiac function are limited (61). Changes in heart structure and function that can lead to HF and atrial fibrillation are the effects of T2DM and obesity on circulation (including vascular function and heart valves) (62).

The aim of our study was to investigate the relationship between MetS parameters and LV functions, using color tissue Dopplerography and 2D speckle-tracking method (2D-STI).

Methods

Fifty patients with MetS who met the diagnostic criteria of MetS of the International Diabetes Federation (IDF) were included in the study. All subjects underwent an echocardiographic study with evaluation of global systolic and diastolic function parameters of the left ventricle. Qlab online analysis software was used to analyze each group, including GLS determination.

Results

- *E/A* ratios varied from 0.4 to 1.7 (average, 0.76) (Figure 4.1).
- Values of septal *é/á* between studies ranged from 0.4 to 0.8 (average, 0.65) (Table 4.5).
- The values of lateral *é/á* between studies varied from 0.5 to 1.9 (mean, 0.89).
- MAPSE values between studies varied from 8.6 to 19.4 (mean, 14.47).
- TAPSE values between studies varied from 15.2 to 30.9 (mean, 22.25).
- GLS values across studies ranged from −11.7% to −23% (mean, 16.8%).
- MD values between studies varied from 3.4 to 62.5 (mean, 22.54).
- Septal *ś* values between studies varied from 5.4 to 10.2 (mean, 7.89).
- Lateral *ś* values between studies varied from 5.9 to 15.9 (mean, −8.7).
- EF values varied from 52% to 60% (mean, 56.47%).
- The age of the patients varied from 52 to 60 years (average age, −52); female −18 (36%), male 32 (64%).

Table 4.5 Echocardiographic Parameters of MetS ($N = 50$)

Factor	Mean ± SD	p value
Age	52 ± 10	
E/A velocity ratio	0.76 ± 0.21	<0.00001
Septal é/á	0.65 ± 0.1	<0.00001
Lateral é/á	0.89 ± 0.28	<0.00001
MAPSE	14.47 ± 3.26	<0.00001
TAPSE	22.25 ± 3.85	<0.00001
EF	56.47 ± 2.2	0.0023
GLS	−16.8 ± 2.53	<0.00001
MD	22.54 ± 16.04	0.04
Septal ś	7.89 ± 1.47	<0.00001
Lateral ś	8.7 ± 2.14	<0.00001

Note: p value significant at <0.05.
Abbreviation: SD, standard deviation.

Conclusion

- MetS has an impact on the functional state of the heart.
- MetS does not decrease LV systolic function—EF, MAPSE, worsening.
- MetS does not cause deterioration of RV systolic function: TAPSE.
- MetS does not cause deterioration of the mechanical dispersion index (MD).
- MetS does not cause a decrease in mean septal ś.
- MetS causes a decrease in LV diastolic function (mean E/A).
- MetS causes a mean septal é/á decrease.
- MetS causes a decrease in average lateral é/á.
- MetS causes a decrease in mean lateral ś.
- MetS causes a decrease in mean GLS.
- 2D STE and tissue Doppler can be used as a reliable method for early detection of LV myocardial damage in patients with MetS.
- Further studies are needed to develop specific therapies that may be more effective in the prevention and treatment of MetS-induced cardiac changes.

5 Discussion of Results Obtained

At different stages of the research, we conducted echocardiographic research on 250 individuals, 50 of whom were healthy and made up the control group.

The study was carried out on a PHILIPS expert-class device Epiq-7.

The echocardiographic study included the use of standard methods and the study of the closest parameters according to the guidelines of the American Society of Echocardioscopy (ASE) and the European Cardiovascular Association (EACVI) (23).

Due to the scarce data on the issue in the literature, at different stages of the research, we conducted a study of individual parameters and compared them with the data in the literature.

During the research process, the following were studied at different stages:

Normal parameters of *LV* mechanical dispersion determined by 2D longitudinal strain speckle-tracking method in healthy subjects

During the study, 50 healthy adult subjects with normal diastolic function and normal EF were prospectively studied.

The results obtained are consistent with the data available in the literature.

DOI: 10.1201/9781003433019-5

If tissue Doppler é/á ratio of the *LV* septal wall has additional diagnostic value in the assessment of *LV* diastolic dysfunction

According to the data available in the literature, there are changes in individual indicators of diastolic function during MetS.

At the same time, the correlation of color tissue Dopplerography indicators with diastolic function has not been established.

We prospectively studied 50 adults (27 men, 23 women, mean age 59 ± 14 years) with mild diastolic dysfunction (class I) and normal LVEF.

During the study, the ratio of the early diastolic speed *é* of the LV septal wall to the late diastolic speed *á* was studied in patients with mild diastolic dysfunction, which was found to be decreased compared to the norm for this parameter. The result obtained can become the basis of a large-scale study, the purpose of which will be to determine the specified *é/á* parameter in patients with different degrees of diastolic dysfunction—mild-relaxation disorder, moderate-pseudo-normal, severe-restrictive—and its correlation with diastolic function as a result.

Values of *LV* septal-lateral early and late tissue Doppler velocity ratio in subjects with normal diastolic function

Because contemporary guidelines on the management of diastolic dysfunction are open to debate, finding an appropriate technique to determine the normal parameters of relatively new echocardiographic parameters remains relevant.

We prospectively studied 50 adult subjects, with normal diastolic function and normal LVEF. LV septal-lateral early and late tissue Doppler velocity ratios were evaluated, which were consistent with the results of a single study in the literature.

GLS in patients with mild diastolic dysfunction and normal EF

Longitudinal strain rates in patients with diastolic dysfunction have not been established. We studied 48 patients with mild diastolic dysfunction, of which 39 were women and 9 were men.

The results obtained indicate a correlation between global longitudinal tension and mild heart diastolic dysfunction.

Echocardiographic parameters of MetS

In the final stage of our study, we studied 10 echocardiographic parameters in patients with MetS, which are not described in the medical literature we reviewed; this confirms the significance of our study.

Fifty patients with MetS who met the diagnostic criteria of MetS of the International Diabetes Federation (IDF) were included in the study. The online Qlab analysis software was used to analyze each group including GLS determination.

Case 1

Male, 56 years old

BMI: 32.76, blood pressure: 207/101 mmHg; HDL cholesterol: 0.91 mmol/L ($N \geq 1.55$); low-density lipoprotein: 3.34 mmol/L (<2.59), TRIGL: 2.82($N < 2.26$ mmol/L)

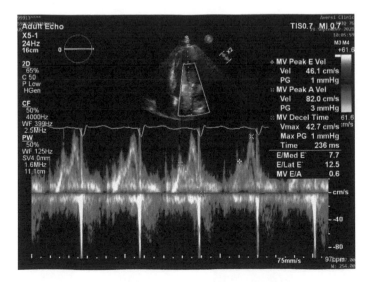

Figure 5.1 The ratio of early and late diastolic velocities of transmitral flow: *E/A*-0.6 ($N > 0.9$).

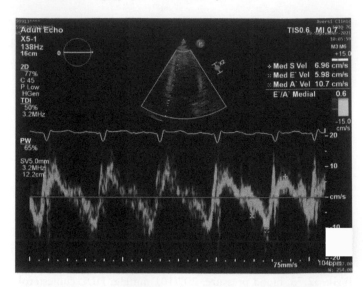

Figure 5.2 The ratio of early and late diastolic velocities determined by color tissue Doppler of the septal wall: *É/Á* 0.6 (*N* > 1).

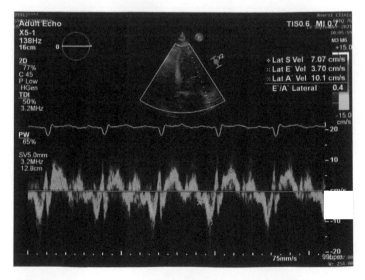

Figure 5.3 The ratio of early and late diastolic velocities determined by color tissue Doppler of the lateral wall: *É/Á* 0.4 (*N* > 1).

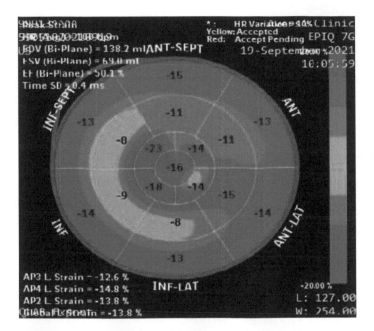

Figure 5.4 GLS: –13.8% (N = –20%).

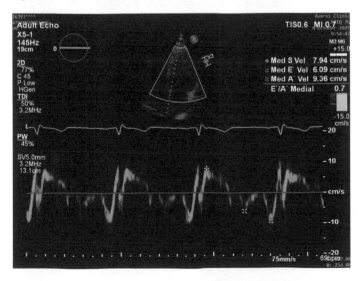

Figure 5.5 The ratio of early and late diastolic velocities determined by color tissue Doppler of the septal wall: *É/A'* med-0.7 (N > 1).

Case 2

Male, 52 years
GLUC: 8.30 mmol/L, HDL cholesterol: 1.29, TRIGL: 2.38, blood
   pressure: 148/78 mmHg, cm 37

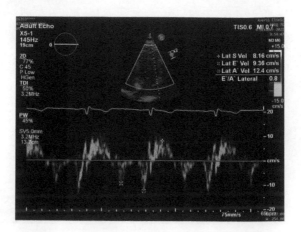

Figure 5.6 The ratio of early and late diastolic velocities determined by
   color tissue Doppler of the lateral wall: *É/Á* lat-0.8 (*N* > 1).

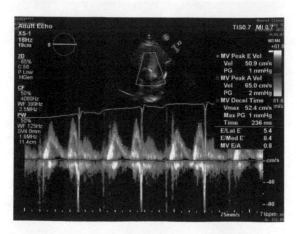

Figure 5.7 The ratio of early and late diastolic velocities of the transmitral flow: *E/A*-0.8 (*N* > 0.9).

Decreased segmental strain: mid-inferior-septal and basal-anterior-septal (blue areas)

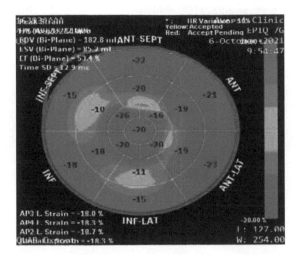

Figure 5.8 GLS: −18.38% (N = −20%).

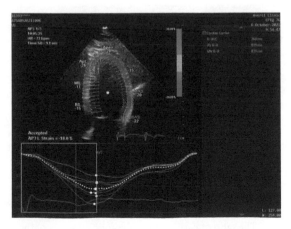

Figure 5.9 Vector direction of endocardial-myocardial-epicardial fibers in patients with MetS.

Case 3

Male, 50 years

GLUC: 6.99 mmol/L, HDL cholesterol: 1.17 mmol/L, TRIG: 1.14
   mmol/L, blood pressure: 150/90 mmHg, BMI: 42

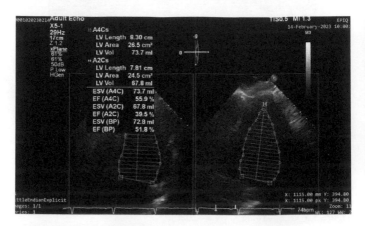

Figure 5.10 Normal EF: 51.8%.

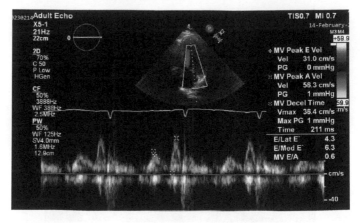

Figure 5.11 The ratio of early and late diastolic velocities of the transmitral flow: -*E/A*-0.6.

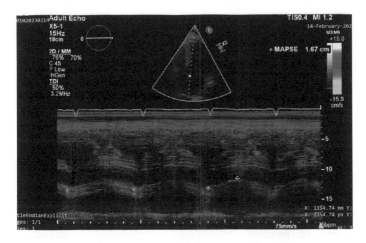

Figure 5.12 Mitral annular peak systolic excursion: 16.7 mm.

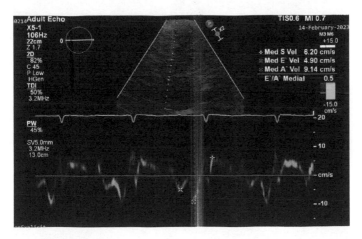

Figure 5.13 Septal *é/á*: 0.5.

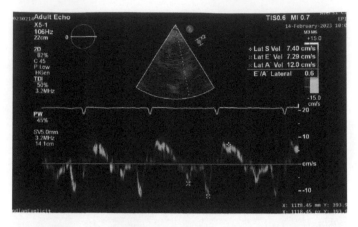

Figure 5.14 Lateral *é/á*: –0.6.

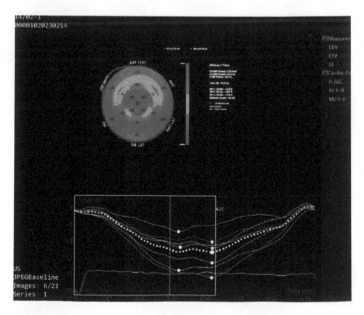

Figure 5.15 GLS, –16.5% (decreased).

Decreased Segmental Strain

The cases we analyzed confirm the results of our study of changes in echocardiographic parameters during MetS; in particular, we noted a decrease in the ratio of transmitral early and late diastolic velocities (*E/A*), a decrease in the ratio of early and late diastolic velocities determined by tissue Doppler echocardiography (*é/á*), and a decrease in the GLS and segmental strain.

1. GLS in patients with mild diastolic dysfunction and normal EF (*N* = 48)
2. Normal indicators of LV mechanical dispersion determined by 2D longitudinal strain speckle-tracking method in healthy subjects (*N* = 50)

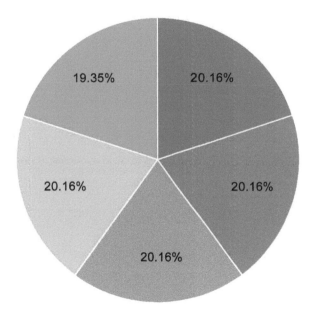

Figure 5.16 Distribution of subjects involved in the study.

3. Indicators of LV septal-lateral early and late tissue Doppler velocity ratio in subjects with normal diastolic function ($N = 50$)

4. Does the tissue Doppler *é/á* ratio of the LV septal wall have additional diagnostic value in the assessment of LV diastolic dysfunction? ($N = 50$)

5. Echocardiographic parameters of MetS ($N = 50$)

6 Conclusions

We conclude that it is realistic to consider the idea of MetS risk stratification, which will significantly contribute to the improvement of the MetS management strategy, taking into account the combination of risk factors.

- Structural and functional changes of the heart are observed during MetS.
- MetS does not cause deterioration of the global systolic function (EF) of the left ventricle in patients without CAD.
- MetS leads to deterioration of LV diastolic function.
- During MetS, there is a decrease in the ratio of early and late diastolic velocity of the septal-lateral walls of the left ventricle.
- MetS leads to a decrease in GLS.
- During MetS, in the case of normal GLS, there is a decrease in regional longitudinal strain.
- Mild diastolic dysfunction is correlated with decreased GLS.

DOI: 10.1201/9781003433019-6

7 Practical Recommendations

- Separation of the risk group from the general population for the purpose of early diagnosis of MetS and subsequent targeted screening
- Focusing the attention of practicing physicians on the manifestation of MetS in the pre-clinical period
- To the extent that the remodeling of the left ventricle is reversible up to a certain stage, continuous monitoring instituted as soon as the first signs of structural-functional changes appear, by taking timely treatment measures and echocardiographic control
- Continuous monitoring of individuals at high risk for MetS without structural heart damage and structural heart damage without clinical manifestation of HF
- Special attention to the manifestation of asymptomatic diastolic dysfunction of the left ventricle in the risk group (without clinical manifestation of MetS) and implementation of timely therapeutic measures and continuous monitoring
- Evaluation and monitoring of GLS and tissue Dopplerography indicators during the course of MetS
- Timely implementation of anti-modeling measures and initiation of treatment at an early stage in patients with MetS
- Planning of studies of the molecular mechanisms of MetS and its genetic disposition, as the early manifestations of cardiac remodeling are related to the delicate events taking place in cardiomyocytes, as well as of indicators of diastolic HF, deformation, tissue Doppler echocardiography, and mechanical dispersion
- Lifestyle changes to prevent MetS: weight reduction, physical activity, alcohol restriction, salt restriction, increased vegetable and fruit consumption, low-fat food consumption

DOI: 10.1201/9781003433019-7

References

1. Detection and management of metabolic syndrome in general medical practice National recommendation of clinical practice (guideline) was approved by the order of the Minister of Health and Social Protection of August 16, 2010 N256/o.
2. Dutka R, Chmir N, Svitlik G, Leontieva S. Prolactin, cortisol, free thyroxine and thyrotropin hormone as risk factors for ischemic heart disease and type-2 diabetes-metabolic syndrome stage marker. *Georgian Med. News*. 2020;3(300).
3. Avaghimian A, Sukasian L, Saakian K, Gevorgian T, Aznaurian A. Molecular mechanisms of cardiovascular homeostasis disorders induced by diabetes (overview). *Georgian Med. News*. 2021;6(315).
4. Chumburidze N, Kezel T, Avaliani Z, Mirziashvili M, Avaliani T, Gongadze N. Relationship between type 2 diabetes and tuberculosis. *Georgian Med. News*. 2020;300:69–74.
5. Biennial Collaborative Agreement (BCA) between the Ministry of Labour, Health and Social Affairs of Georgia and the Regional Office for Europe of the World Health Organisation. *Summary Report*. Risk Factor Survey; 2007.
6. International Diabetes Federation. *IDF Diabetes Atlas*. 9th ed. Brussels: International Diabetes Federation; 2019.
7. 2019 ESC guidelines on diabetes, pre-diabetes, and cardiovascular diseases developed in collaboration with the EASD. *Eur. Heart J*. 2020;41(2):255–323. https://doi.org/10.1093/eurheartj/ehz486 .
8. Grundy SM, et al. Diagnosis and management of the metabolic syndrome: An American Heart Association/National Heart, Lung and Blood Institute scientific statement. *Circulation*. 2005;112(17): 2735–2752.
9. Perrone-Filardi P, et al. The role of metabolic syndrome in heart failure. *Eur. Heart J*. 2015;36(39):2015–2036.
10. Purwowiyoto SL, Prawara AS. Metabolic syndrome and heart failure: Mechanism and management. *Med. Pharm. Rep*. 2021;94(1): 15–21.

11. Dos Santosa LRB, Fleminga I. Role of cytochrome P450-derived, polyunsaturated fatty acid mediators in diabetes and the metabolic syndrome. *Prostaglandins Other Lipid Mediat.* 2020;148:106407.

12. Luís C, Fernandes R, Soaresa R, von Hafed P. A state of the art review on the novel mediator asprosin in the metabolic syndrome. *Porto Biomed. J.* 2020;5(6):e108.

13. Teixeira PFDS, dos Santos PB, Pazos-Moura CC. The role of thyroid hormone in metabolism and metabolic syndrome. *Ther. Adv. Endocrinol. Metab.* 2020;11:1–33.

14. Satoh T, Wang L, Levine A, Baust J, Wyman S, Wu Y, Watkins C, McTiernan CF, Gladwin MT. Metabolic syndrome contributes to the pulmonary arterial dysfunction in pulmonary hypertension in heart failure with preserved ejection fraction. *Eur. Heart J.* 2020;41.

15. Kasahara T, Endoh S, Ohtahara A, Kawatani S, Amisaki R, Mizuta E, Adachi M, Osaki S. The inverse association between lipoprotein(a) levels and metabolic syndorome and its components on coronary artery disease patients. *Eur. Heart J.* 2020;41.

16. von Korn P, Kia S, Lechner K, Dinges S, Duvinage A, Scherr J, Landmesser U, Halle M, Kraenkel N. Inter-individual differences in the response to an exercise training intervention in patients with metabolic syndrome. *Clin. Res. Cardiol.* 2020;109(Suppl 1):Beitrag V265.

17. Hu Y, Zhu Y, Lian N, Chen M, Bartke A, Yuan R. Metabolic syndrome and skin diseases. *Front. Endocrinol.* 2019;10:788. https://doi.org/10.3389/fendo.2019.00788.

18. Dong S, Wang Z, Shen K, Chen X. Metabolic syndrome and breast cancer: Prevalence, treatment response, and prognosis. *Front. Oncol.* 2021;11:62966.

19. Lotti F, Marchiani S, Corona G, Maggi M. Metabolic syndrome and reproduction. *Int. J. Mol. Sci.* 2021;22:1988. https://doi.org/10.3390/ijms22041988.

20. Lillich FF, Imig JD, Proschak E. Multi-target approaches in metabolic syndrome. *Front. Pharmacol.* 2021;11:554961. https://doi.org/10.3389/fphar.2020.554961.

21. Yamase Y, Horibe H, Kato K, Oguri M, Fujimaki T, Hibino T, Kondo T, Sakuma J, Takeuchi I, Murohara T, Yasukochi Y, Yamada Y. Identification of four genes as novel susceptibility loci for early-onset type 2 diabetes mellitus, metabolic syndrome, or hyperuricemia. *Biomed. Rep.* 2018;9(1):21–36.

22. Bansal R, Gubbi S, Muniyappa R. Metabolic syndrome and COVID 19: Endocrine-immune-vascular interactions shapes clinical course. *Endocrinology.* 2020;161(10):bqaa112.

23. Yanai H. Metabolic syndrome and COVID 19: Endocrine-immune-vascular interactions shapes clinical course. *Cardiol. Res.* 2020;11(6):360–365.

24. Perez-Galarza JM, Muka T, Baldeon LY, Freire WB, Drexhage HA, Franco OH. Prevalence of overweight, obesity and metabolic syndrome among adult Ecuadorian population: The ENSANUT study. *Eur. Heart J.* 2017;38:914–915.

25. La Sala L, Pontiroli AE. Review prevention of diabetes and cardiovascular disease in obesity. *Int. J. Mol. Sci.* 2020;21(21):8178. https://doi.org/10.3390/ijms21218178.

26. Bao Y, Lu J, Wang C, et al. Obesity, metabolic syndrome and bariatric surgery: A narrative review. *J. Diabetes Investig.* 2020;11(2):294–296.

27. Kwon CH, et al. Impact of metabolic syndrome on the incidence of atrial fibrillation: A nationwide longitudinal cohort study in South Korea. *J. Clin. Med.* 2019;8(8):1095.

28. Katbeh A, De Potter T, Geelen P, Balogh Z, Stefanidis E, Iliodromitis K, Barbato E, Van Camp G, Penicka M. The effect of hypertension and metabolic syndrome on left atrial function in patients with paroxysmal atrial fibrillation undergoing catheter ablation. *Eur. Heart J.* 2019;40(Suppl 1).

29. Goncalves Teixeira PM, Ladeiras Lopes R, Bettencourt P, Azevedo A, Leite-Moreira A, Fontes-Carvalho R. Metabolic syndrome severity score is a predictor of worse diastolic function independently of each individual metabolic syndrome component: A community-based cohort study. *Eur. Heart J.* 2018;39(Suppl 1).

30. Ivanovic B, et al. The influence of isolated metabolic syndrome, diabetes and hypertension on right ventricular structure and function. *Eur. Heart J.* 2013;34(Suppl 1):4147.

31. Lee JB, et al. Components of metabolic syndrome are associated with diastolic dysfunction. *Eur. Heart J.* 2015;36

32. Donohue A, et al. Echocardiographic measures of systolic and diastolic function as predictors of incident heart failure in metabolic syndrome and diabetes. *JACC.* 2011;57:E274.

33. Wang Q, et al. Two-dimensional speckle tracking imaging in evaluating clinical of left ventricular myocardial lesions in patients with metabolic syndrome. *JACC.* 2015;66.

34. La Carruba S, et al. Left ventricular dysfunction and metabolic syndrome in hospitalized patients. *Eur. J. Echocardiogr.* 2006;7(Suppl 1):S124.

35. Parapid B, et al. The metabolic syndrome and coronary heart disease: 40—years in the Seven Countries Study. *EHJ.* 2015;36.

36. Kosmala W, Sanders P, Marwick TH. Subclinical myocardial impairment in metabolic diseases. *JACC: Cardiovasc. Imaging.* 2017;10(6): 692–703.

37. Guembe MJ, Fernandez-Lazaro CI, Sayon-Orea C, Toledo E, Moreno-Iribas C, RIVANA Study Investigators. Risk for cardiovascular disease associated with metabolic syndrome and its components:

A 13-year prospective study in the RIVANA cohort. *Cardiovasc. Diabetol.* 2020;19(1):195.

38. Roth GA, Abate D, Abate KH, Abay SM, Abbafati C, et al. Global, regional, and national age-sex-specifc mortality for 282 causes of death in 195 countries and territories, 1980–2017: A systematic analysis for the Global Burden of Disease Study 2017. *Lancet.* 2018;392:1736–1788.

39. Kyu HH, Abate D, Abate KH, Abay SM, Abbafati C, Abbasi N, et al. Global, regional, and national disability-adjusted life-years (DALYs) for 359 diseases and injuries and healthy life expectancy (HALE) for 195 countries and territories, 1990–2017: A systematic analysis for the Global Burden of Disease Study 2017. *Lancet.* 2018;392:1859–1922.

40. Wilkins E, Wilson L, Wickramasinghe K, Bhatnagar P, Leal J, Luengo-Fernandez R, et al. *European Cardiovascular Disease Statistics 2017.* Brussels: European Heart Network; 2017. https://researchportal.bath.ac.uk/en/publications/european-cardiovascular-disease-statistics-2017. Accessed 1 March 2020.

41. Simmons RK, Alberti KGMM, Gale EAM, Colagiuri S, Tuomilehto J, Qiao Q, et al. The metabolic syndrome: Useful concept or clinical tool? Report of a WHO expert consultation. *Diabetologia.* 2010;53:600–605.

42. Alberti KGMM, Eckel RH, Grundy SM, Zimmet PZ, Cleeman JI, Donato KA, et al. Harmonizing the metabolic syndrome: A joint interim statement of the International Diabetes Federation Task Force on Epidemiology and Prevention; National Heart, Lung, and Blood Institute; American Heart Association; World Heart Federation; International Atherosclerosis Society; and International Association for the Study of Obesity. *Circulation.* 2009;120:1640–1645.

43. Mendrick DL, Diehl AM, Topor LS, Dietert RR, Will Y, La Merrill MA, Bouret S, Varma V, Hastings KL, Schug TT. Metabolic syndrome and associated diseases: From the bench to the clinic. *J. Annals Mae Diehl.* 2015.

44. Bouret SG. Organizational actions of metabolic hormones. *Front. Neuroendocrinol.* 2013;34:18–26.

45. Bray MS, Loos RJ, McCaffery JM, Ling C, Franks PW, Weinstock GM, Snyder MP, Vassy JL, AgursCollins T. NIH working group report-using genomic information to guide weight management: From universal to precision treatment. *Obesity (Silver Spring).* 2016;24:14–22.

46. Locke AE, Kahali B, Berndt SI, Justice AE, Pers TH, Day FR, Powell C, Vedantam S, Buchkovich ML, Yang J, et al. Genetic studies of body mass index yield new insights for obesity biology. *Nature.* 2015;518:197–206.

47. Lumeng CN. Innate immune activation in obesity. *Mol. Aspects Med.* 2013;34:12–29.
48. Henao-Mejia J, Elinav E, Jin C, Hao L, Mehal WZ, Strowig T, Thaiss CA, Kau AL, Eisenbarth SC, Jurczak MJ, et al. Inflammasome-mediated dysbiosis regulates progression of NAFLD and obesity. *Nature.* 2012;482:179–185.
49. Maes et al.; Stunkard et al. BMI; 1997.
50. Lemieux I, Després J-P. Metabolic syndrome past, present and future. *Nutrients.* 2020;12:3501. https://doi.org/10.3390/nu12113501.
51. Yates KF, Sweat V, Yau PL, Turchiano MM, Convit A. Impact of metabolic syndrome on cognition and brain: A selected review of the literature. *Arterioscler. Thromb. Vasc. Biol.* 2012;32:2060–2067.
52. Avgerinos KI, Spyrou N, Mantzoros CS, Dalamaga M. Obesity and cancer risk: Emerging biological mechanisms and perspectives. *Metabolism.* 2019;92:121–135.
53. Després JP. Predicting longevity using metabolomics: A novel tool for precision lifestyle medicine? *Nat. Rev. Cardiol.* 2020;17:67–68.
54. Rodriges-Zanella H, Boccalini F, et al. Left ventricular mechanical dispersion measured with two-dimensional speckle tracking echocardiography predicts severe arrhythmic events in patients with ischemic and nonishemic cardiomyopathy. *Eur. Heart J.* 2017;18.
55. Hensen LCR, Goossens K, Podlesnikar T, Rotmans JI, Jukema JW, Delgado V, Bax JJ. Left ventricular mechanical dispersion and global longitudinal strain and ventricular arrhythmias in predialysis and dialysis patients. *Eur. Heart J. Cardiovasc. Imaging.* 2019;20.
56. Aagaard EN, Kvisvik B, Pervez MO, Lyngbakken MN, Berge T, Enger S, Orstad EB, Smith P, Omland T, Tveit A, Røsjø H, Steine K. Left ventricular dispersion in a general population: Data from Akershus Cardiac Examination, 1950 study. *Eur. Heart J. Cardiovasc. Imaging.* 2020;21(2):183–190.
57. Hill JC, Palma RA.
58. Hill JC, Palma RA. Doppler tissue imaging for the assesment of left ventricular diastolic function: A systematic approach for the sono graphers. *J. Am. Soc. Echocardiogr.* 2005;18(1):80–88.
59. Kou S, Caballero L, Dulgheru R, Henri C, Bensahi I, Elfhal A, Ferro G, Lanceloti P. Differences in tissue doppler imaging parametres of left ventricular systolic function according to gender and age in healthy subjects. *Eur. Heart J.* 2014;35.
60. Nikitin NP, Witte KKA, Thackray SDR, de Silva R, Clark AL, Cleland JGF. Longitudinal ventricular function: Normal values of atrioventricular annular and myocardial velocities measured with quantitative two-dimensional color doppler tissue imaging. *J. Am. Soc. Echocardiogr.* 2003;16(9):906–921.

61. Rodríguez-Zanella H, Haugaa K, Boccalini F, Secco E, Edvardsen T, Badano LP, Muraru D. Physiological determinants of left ventricular mechanical dispersion: A 2-dimensional speckle tracking echocardiographic study in healthy volunteer. *JACC: Cardiovasc. Imaging.* 2018;11(4):648–645.

62. Lee JB, Hong SP, Lee YS, Jk RYU, Choi JY, Kim KS, Son JH, Park YW, Kim BK, Lee CW. Components of metabolic syndrome are associated with diastolic dysfunction. *Republic Eur. Heart J.* 2015;36:118.

63. Sanders P, Marwick TH.Subclinical myocardial impairment in metabolic diseases. *JACC: Cardiovasc. Imaging.* 2017;10(6):2017.

64. Lakka HM, Laaksonen DE, Lakka TA, et al. The metabolic syndrome and total and cardiovascular disease mortality in middle-aged men. *JAMA.* 2002;288:2709–2716.

65. Isomaa B, Almgren P, Tuomi T, et al. Cardiovascular morbidity and mortality associated with the metabolic syndrome. *Diabetes Care.* 2001;24:683–689.

66. Malik S, Wong ND, Franklin SS, et al. The impact of the metabolic syndrome on mortality from coronary heart disease, cardiovascular disease, and all causes in United States adults. *Circulation.* 2004;110:1239–1244.

67. Voigt J-U, Pedrizzetti G, Lysyansky P, Marwick TH, Houle H, Baumann R, Pedri S, Ito Y, Abe Y, Metz S, Song JH, Hamilton J, Sengupta PP, Kolias TJ, d'Hooge J, Aurigemma GP, Thomas JD, Badano LP. Definitions for a common standard for 2D speckletracking echocardiography: Consensus document of the EACVI/ASE/Industry Task Force to standardize deformation imaging. *Eur. Heart J.—Cardiovasc. Imaging.* 2015;16:1–11. https://doi.org/10.1093/ehjci/jeu184

68. Geyer H, Caracciolo G, Abe H, Wilansky S, Carerj S, Gentile F, et al. Assessment of myocardial mechanics using speckle tracking echocardiography: fundamentals and clinical applications. *J. Am. Soc. Echocardiogr.* 2010;23:351–369.

69. Mondillo S, Galderisi M, Mele D, Cameli M, Lomoriello VS, Zaca' V, et al. Speckle tracking echocardiography: A new technique for assessing myocardial function. *J. Ultrasound Med.* 2011;30:71–83.

70. Haugaa KH, Smedsrud MK, Steen T, Kongsgaard E, Loennechen JP, Skjaerpe T, et al. Mechanical dispersion assessed by myocardial strain in patients after myocardial infarction for risk prediction of ventricular arrhythmia. *JACC Cardiovasc. Imaging.* 2010;3:247–256.

71. Haugaa KH, Hasselberg NE, Edvardsen T. Mechanical dispersion by strain echocardiography: A predictor of ventricular arrhyth. *Eur. Heart J.—Cardiovasc. Imaging.* 2015;16:1000–1007. https://doi.org/10.1093/ehjci/jev027

72. Rubler S, Dlugash J, Yuceoglu YZ, Kumral T, Branwood AW, Grishman A. New type of cardiomyopathy associated with diabetic glomerulosclerosis. *Am. J. Cardiol.* 1972;30:595–602.

73. Poirier P, Bogaty P, Garneau C, Marois L, Dumesnil JG. Diastolic dysfunction in normotensive men with well-controlled type 2 diabetes: Importance of maneuvers in echocardiographic screening for preclinical diabetic cardiomyopathy. *Diabetes Care*. 2001;24:5–10.
74. Boudina S, Abel ED. Diabetic cardiomyopathy revisited. *Circulation*. 2007;115:3213–3223.
75. Spector KS. Diabetic cardiomyopathy. *Clin. Cardiol.* 1998;21:885–887.
76. Tziakas DN, Chalikias GK, Kaski JC. Epidemiology of the diabetic heart. *Coron. Artery Dis.* 2005;16(Suppl. 1):S3–S10.
77. Curtis JP, Sokol SI, Wang Y, Rathore SS, Ko DT, Jadbabaie F, et al. The association of left ventricular ejection fraction, mortality, and cause of death in stable outpatients with heart failure. *J. Am. Coll. Cardiol.* 2003;42:736–742.
78. Otterstad JE, Froeland G, St John Sutton M, Holme I. Accuracy and reproducibility of biplane two-dimensional echocardiographic measurements of left ventricular dimensions and function. *Eur. Heart J.* 1997;18:507–513.
79. Marwick TH. Methods used for the assessment of LV systolic function: Common currency or tower of Babel? *Heart.* 2013;99:1078–1086.
80. Thomas JD, Popovic ZB. Assessment of left ventricular function by cardiac ultrasound. *J. Am. Coll. Cardiol.* 2006;48:2012–2025.
81. Amundsen BH, Helle-Valle T, Edvardsen T, Torp H, Crosby J, Lyseggen E, et al. Noninvasive myocardial strain measurement by speckle tracking echocardiography: Validation against sonomicrometry and tagged magnetic resonance imaging. *J. Am. Coll. Cardiol.* 2006;47:789–793.
82. Mignot A, Donal E, Zaroui A, Reant P, Salem A, Hamon C, et al. Global longitudinal strain as a major predictor of cardiac events in patients with depressed left ventricular function: A multicenter study. *J. Am. Soc. Echocardiogr.* 2010;23:1019–1024.
83. Nahum J, Bensaid A, Dussault C, Macron L, Clemence D, Bouhemad B, et al. Impact of longitudinal myocardial deformation on the prognosis of chronic heart failure patients. *Circ. Cardiovasc. Imaging.* 2010;3:249–256.
84. Iacoviello M, Puzzovivo A, Guida P, Forleo C, Monitillo F, Catanzaro R, et al. Independent role of left ventricular global longitudinal strain in predicting prognosis of chronic heart failure patients. *Echocardiography.* 2013;30:803–811.
85. Cho GY, Marwick TH, Kim HS, Kim MK, Hong KS, Oh DJ. Global 2-dimensional strain as a new prognosticator in patients with heart failure. *J. Am. Coll. Cardiol.* 2009;54.
86. Srivastavaa M, Burrella LM, Calafioreb P. Lateral vs medial mitral annular tissue Doppler in the echocardiographic assessment of diastolic function and filling pressures: Which should we use? *Eur. J. Echocardiogr.* 2005;6:97e106.

87. Farias CA, Rodriguez L, Garcia MJ, Sun JP, Klein AL, Thomas JD. Assessment of diastolic function by tissue Doppler echocardiography: Comparison with standard transmitral and pulmonary venous flow. *J. Am. Soc. Echocardiogr.* 1999;12:609e17.

88. Waggoner AD, Bierig SM. Tissue Doppler imaging: A useful echocardiographic method for the cardiac sonographer to assess systolic and diastolic ventricular function. *J. Am. Soc. Echocardiogr.* 2001;14:1143e52.

89. Garcia MJ, Thomas JD. Tissue Doppler to assess diastolic left ventricular function. *Echocardiography.* 1999;16:501e8.

90. Sohn DW, Chai IH, Lee DJ, Kim HC, Kim HS, Oh BH, et al. Assessment of mitral annulus velocity by Doppler tissue imaging in the evaluation of left ventricular diastolic function. *J. Am. Coll. Cardiol.* 1997;30:474e80.

91. Ommen SR, Nishimura RA, Appleton CP, Miller FA, Oh JK, Redfield MM, et al. Clinical utility of Doppler echocardiography and tissue Doppler imaging in the estimation of left ventricular filling pressures: A comparative simultaneous Doppler-catheterization study. *Circulation.* 2000;102:1788e94.

92. Nishimura RA, Appleton CP, Redfield MM, Ilstrup DM, Holmes Jr. DR, Tajik AJ. Noninvasive Doppler echocardiographic evaluation of left ventricular filling pressures in patients with cardiomyopathies: A simultaneous Doppler echocardiographic and cardiac catheterization study. *J. Am. Coll. Cardiol.* 1996;28:1226e33.

93. Nagueh SF, Mikati I, Kopelen HA, Middleton KJ, Quinones MA, Zoghbi WA. Doppler estimation of left ventricular filling pressure in sinus tachycardia. A new application of tissue Doppler imaging. *Circulation.* 1998;98:1644e50.

94. Mitchell C, Rahko PS, Blauwet LA, Canaday B, Finstuen JA, Foster MC, Horton K, Ogunyankin KO, Palma RA, Velazquez EJ. Guidelines for performing a comprehensive transthoracic echocardiographic examination in adults: Recommendations from the American society of echocardiography. *J. Am.Soc. Echocardiogr.* 2019;32(1):1–64.

95. Brown LM, Duffy CE, Mitchell C, Young L. A practical guide to pediatric coronary artery imaging with echocardiography. *J. Am. Soc. Echocardiogr.* 2015;28:379–391.

96. Garcia MJ, Smedira NG, Greenberg NL, Main M, Firstenberg MS, Odabashian J, et al. Color M-mode Doppler flow propagation velocity is a preload insensitive index of left ventricular relaxation: Animal and human validation. *J. Am. Coll. Cardiol.* 2000;35:201–208.

97. Nagueh SF, Smiseth OA, Appleton CP, Byrd BF, Dokainish H, Edvardsen T, Flachskampf FA, Gillebert TC, Klein AL, Lancellotti P, Marino P, Oh JK, Popescu BA, Waggoner AD. Recommendations for the evaluation of left ventricular diastolic function by echocardiography: An update from the american society of echocardiography and the European association of cardiovascular imaging. *J. Am. Soc. Echocardiogr.* 2016;29:277–314.

98. Wu M-Z, Chen Y, Zou Y, Zhen Z, Yu Y-J, Liu Y-X, Yuen M, Ho L-M, Lam KS-L, Tse H-F, Yiu K-H. Impact of obesity on longitudinal changes tocardiac structure and function in patients with Type 2 diabetes mellitus. *Eur. Heart J.—Cardiovasc. Imaging.* 2019;20.

99. Scherrer-Crosbie M. *Heart Imaging in Obesity, Metabolic Syndrome and Diabetes: Similarities and Differences.* EuroEcho; 2015.

100. Ponikowski P, et al. 2016 ESC Guidelines for the diagnosis and treatment of acute and chronic heart failure. *Eur. Heart J.* 2016; 37:2129–2200.

101. Zamorano JL, et al. 2016 ESC Position Paper on cancer treatments and cardiovascular toxicity developed under the auspices of the ESC committee for practice guidelines. *Eur. Heart J.* 2016;37.

102. Marwick TH. Brisbane Measurement of strain and strain rate by echocardiography ready for prime time? *J. Am. Coll. Cardiol.* 2006;47:1313–1327.

103. Yu C-M, Sanderson JE, Marwick TH, Oh JK. Tissue Doppler imaging a new prognosticator for cardiovascular diseases. *J. Am. Coll. Cardiol.* 2007;49(19):1903–1914.

104. Binder T. EuroEcho; 2019.

105. Tsugu T, et al. Echocardiographic reference ranges for normal left ventricular layer-specific strain: Results from the EACVI NORRE study. *Eur. Heart J.—Cardiovasc. Imaging.* 2020;21:896–905. https://doi.org/10.1093/ehjci/jeaa050.

106. Sengupta PP, Korinek J, Belohlavek M, Narula J. Left ventricular structure and function: Basic science for cardiac imaging. *JACC.* 2006;48(10):1988–2001.

107. Sengupta PP, Tajik AJ, Chandrasekaran K, Khandheria BK. Twist mechanics of the left ventricle principles and application. *JACC Cardiovasc. Imaging.* 2008;1(3):366–376.

108. Cosentino F, et al. 2019 ESC guidelines on diabetes, pre-diabetes, and cardiovascular diseases developed in collaboration with the EASD. *Eur. Heart J.* 2020;41:255323.

109. Williams B, et al. 2018 ESC/ESH guidelines for the management of arterial hypertension. *Eur. Heart J.* 2018;39:3021–3104.

110. Catapano AL. 2016 ESC/EAS guidelines for the management of dyslipidaemias the Task Force for the management of dyslipidaemias of the European Society of Cardiology (ESC) and European Atherosclerosis Society (EAS). *Eur. Heart J.* 2016;37:2999–3058.

112. Duramex G.*How Can Image Guide Treatment in Cardiometabolic Syndrome?* EuroEcho; 2019.

113. Santos-Ferreira D, Ladeiras-Lopes R, Sampaio F, Leite S, Vilela E, Leite-Moreira A, Bettencourt N, Gama V, Braga P, Fontes-Carvalho R. Metformin improves diastolic dysfunction of non-diabetic patients

with metabolic syndrome. The MET-DIME randomized trial. *Endocrine*. 2021;72(3):699–710.

114. Chazova I, Schlaich MP. Improved hypertension control with the imidazoline agonist moxonidine in a multinational metabolic syndrome population: Principal results of the MERSY study. *Int. J. Hypertens*. 2013:Article ID 541689.

115. FIELD study investigators. *Lancet*. 2005;266(9500):1849–1861.

116. Budoff MJ, Raggi P, Beller GA, Berman DS, Druz RS, Malik S, Rigolin VH, Weigold WG, Soman P, On Behalf of the Imaging Council of the American College of Cardiology. Noninvasive cardiovascular risk assessment of the asymptomatic diabetic patient the imaging council of the American college of cardiology. *JACC: Cardiovasc. Imaging*. 2016;9(2).

117. Wang Y, Yang H, Huynh Q, Nolan M, Negishi K, Marwick TH. Diagnosis of nonischemic stage B heart failure in type 2 diabetes mellitus optimal parameters for prediction of heart failure. *JACC: Cardiovasc. Imaging*. 2018;11(10).

118. Ambroselli D, Masciulli F, Romano E, Catanzaro G, Besharat ZM, Massari MC, Ferretti E, Migliaccio S, Izzo L, Ritieni A, Grosso M, Formichi C, Dotta F, Frigerio F, Barbiera E, Giusti AM, Ingallina C, Mannina L. New advances in metabolic syndrome, from prevention to treatment: The role of diet and food. *Nutrients*. 2023;15(3):640.

119. van Veldhuisen SL, Gorter TM, van Woerden G, de Boer RA, Rienstra M, Hazebroek EJ, et al. Bariatric surgery and cardiovascular disease: A systematic review and meta-analysis. *Eur. Heart J*. 2022;43:1955–1969.

120. Bruzzone C, Gil-Redondo R, Seco M, Barragán R, de la Cruz L, Cannet C, Schäfer H, Fang F, Diercks T, Bizkarguenaga M, et al. A molecular signature for the metabolic syndrome by urine metabolomics. *Cardiovasc. Diabetol*. 2021;20:155.

121. Costa FF, Rosário WR, Ribeiro Farias AC, de Souza RG, Duarte Gondim RS, Barroso WA. Metabolic syndrome and COVID-19: An update on the associated comorbidities and proposed therapies. *Diabetes Metab. Syndr. Clin. Res. Rev*. 2020;14:809–814.

122. Pasanta D, Chancharunee S, Tungjai M, Kim HJ, Kothan S. Effects of obesity on the lipid and metabolite profiles of young adults by serum 1H-NMR spectroscopy. *PeerJ*. 2019;7:e7137.

123. Salek RM, Maguire ML, Bentley E, Rubtsov DV, Hough T, Cheeseman M, Nunez D, Sweatman BC, Haselden JN, Cox RD, et al. A metabolomic comparison of urinary changes in type 2 diabetes in mouse, rat, and human. *Physiol. Genom*. 2007;29:99–108.

124. Kim SH, Yang SO, Kim HS, Kim Y, Park T, Choi HK. 1H-nuclear magnetic resonance spectroscopy-based metabolic assessment in

a rat model of obesity induced by a high-fat diet. *Anal. Bioanal. Chem.* 2009;395:1117–1124.

125. Zhang Y, Zhang H, Rong S, Bian C, Yang Y, Pan H. NMR spectroscopy based metabolomics confirms the aggravation of metabolic disorder in metabolic syndrome combined with hyperuricemia. *Nutr. Metab. Cardiovasc. Dis.* 2021;31:2449–2457.

126. Kanbay M, Jensen T, Solak Y, Le M, Roncal-Jimenez C, Rivard C, Lanaspa MA, Nakagawa T, Johnson RJ. Uric acid in metabolic syndrome: From an innocent bystander to a central player. *Eur. J. Intern. Med.* 2016;29:3–8.

127. Bombelli M, Quarti-Trevano F, Tadic M, Facchetti R, Cuspidi C, Mancia G, Grassi G. Uric acid and risk of new-onset metabolic syndrome, impaired fasting glucose and diabetes mellitus in a general Italian population: Data from the Pressioni Arteriose Monitorate e Loro Associazioni study. *J. Hypertens.* 2018;36:1492–1498.

128. Gonzalez-Franquesa A, Burkart AM, Isganaitis E, Patti ME. What have metabolomics approaches taught us about type 2 diabetes? *Curr. Diab. Rep.* 2016;16:74.

129. Hess DA, Verma S, Bhatt D, Bakbak E, Terenzi DC, Puar P, Cosentino F. Vascular repair and regeneration in cardiometabolic diseases. *Eur. Heart J.* 2022;43:450–459. https://doi.org/10.1093/eurheartj/ehab758.

130. Kaptoge S, Pennells L, De Bacquer D, et al. World Health Organization cardiovascular disease risk charts: Revised models to estimate risk in 21 global regions. *Lancet Glob. Health.* 2019;7:e1332–e1345.

131. Herrington W, Lacey B, Sherliker P, Armitage J, Lewington S. Epidemiology of atherosclerosis and the potential to reduce the global burden of atherothrombotic disease. *Circ. Res.* 2016;118:535–546.

132. Roth GA, Abate D, Abate KH, et al. Global, regional, and national age-sex-specific mortality for 282 causes of death in 195 countries and territories, 1980–2017: A systematic analysis for the Global Burden of Disease Study 2017. *Lancet.* 2018;392:1736–1788.

133. Townsend N, Nichols M, Scarborough P, Rayner M. Cardiovascular disease in Europe—Epidemiological update 2015. *Eur Heart J.* 2015;36:2696–2705.

134. Poirier P, Giles TD, Bray GA, et al. Obesity Committee of the Council on Nutrition, Physical Activity, and Metabolism. Obesity and cardiovascular disease: Pathophysiology, evaluation, and effect of weight loss: An update of the 1997 American Heart Association Scientific Statement on obesity and heart disease from the Obesity Committee of the Council on Nutrition, Physical Activity, and Metabolism. *Circulation.* 2006;113:898–918.

135. Bommer C, Heesemann E, Sagalova V, et al. The global economic burden of diabetes in adults aged 20–79 years: A cost-of-illness study. *Lancet Diabetes Endocrinol.* 2017;5:423–430.

136. Solomon SD, McMurray JJV, Claggett B, de Boer RA, DeMets D, Hernandez AF, et al. Dapagliflozin in heart failure with mildly reduced or preserved ejection fraction. *N. Engl. J. Med.* 2022;387:1089–1098.

137. Lavie CJ, Alpert MA, Arena R, Mehra MR, Milani RV, Ventura HO. Impact of obesity and the obesity paradox on prevalence and prognosis in heart failure. *JACC Heart Fail.* 2013;1:93–102.

138. Kalantar-Zadeh K, Block G, Horwich T, Fonarow GC. Reverse epidemiology of conventional cardiovascular risk factors in patients with chronic heart failure. *J. Am. Coll. Cardiol.* 2004;43:1439–1444.

139. Oreopoulos A, Padwal R, Kalantar-Zadeh K, Fonarow GC, Norris CM, McAlister FA. Body mass index and mortality in heart failure: a meta-analysis. *Am. Heart J.* 2008;156:13–22.

140. Gupta PP, Fonarow GC, Horwich TB. Obesity and the obesity paradox in heart failure. *Can. J. Cardiol.* 2015;31:195–202.

141. Fonarow GC, Srikanthan P, Costanzo MR, Cintron GB, Lopatin M for the ADHERE Scientific Advisory Committee and Investigators. An obesity paradox in acute heart failure: Analysis of body mass index and inhospital mortality for 108927 patients in the Acute Decompensated Heart Failure National Registry. *Am. Heart J.* 2007;153:74–81

142. Lavie CJ, Osman AF, Milani RV, Mehra MR. Body composition and prognosis in chronic systolic heart failure: The obesity paradox. *Am. J. Cardiol.* 2003;91:891–894.

143. Perrone-Filardi P, Savarese G, Scaranoc M, Cavazzina R, Trimarco B, Minneci S, Maggioni AP, Tavazzi L, Tognoni G, Marchioli R. Prognostic impact of metabolic syndrome in patients with chronic heart failure: Data from GISSI-HF trial. *Int. J. Cardiol.* 2015;178:85–90.

144. Voulgari C, Tentolouris N, Dilaveris P, Tousoulis D, Katsilambros N, Stefanadis C. Increased heart failure risk in normal-weight people with metabolic syndrome compared with metabolically healthy obese individuals. *J. Am. Coll. Cardiol.* 2011;58:1343–1350.

145. Anker SD, Ponikowski PP, Clark AL, Leyva F, Rauchhaus M, Kemp M, Teixeira MM, Hellewell PG, Hooper J, Poole-Wilson PA, Coats AJ. Cytokines and neurohormones relating to body composition alterations in the wasting syndrome of chronic heart failure. *Eur. Heart J.* 1999;20:683–693.

146. Anker SD, Coats AJ. Cardiac cachexia: A syndrome with impaired survival and immune and neuroendocrine activation. *Chest.* 1999;115:836–847.

147. Anker SD, Negassa A, Coats AJ, Afzal R, Poole-Wilson PA, Cohn JN, Yusuf S. Prognostic importance of weight loss in chronic heart failure and the effect of treatment with angiotensin-converting-enzyme inhibitors: An observational study. *Lancet*. 2003;361:1077–1083.

148. Blair JE, Khan S, Konstam MA, Swedberg K, Zannad F, Burnett JC Jr., Grinfeld L, Maggioni AP, Udelson JE, Zimmer CA, Ouyang J, Chen CF, Gheorghiade M, EVEREST Investigators. Weight changes after hospitalization for worsening heart failure and subsequent rehospitalization and mortality in the EVEREST trial. *Eur. Heart J.* 2009;30:1666–1673.

149. Mottillo S, et al. The metabolic syndrome and cardiovascular risk a systematic review and meta-analysis. *JACC*. 2010;56(14):1113–1132.

150. Tudoran C, Tudoran M, Cut TG, Lazureanu VE, Bende F, Fofiu R, Enache A, Pescariu SA, Novacescu D. The impact of metabolic syndrome and obesity on the evolution of diastolic dysfunction in apparently healthy patients suffering from post-COVID-19 syndrome. *Biomedicines*. 2022;10:1519. https://doi.org/10.3390/biomedicines10071519.

151. Alkhulaifi F, Darkoh C. Meal timing, meal frequency and metabolic syndrome. *Nutrients*. 2022;14:1719. https://doi.org/10.3390/nu14091719.

152. Bauset C, Martínez-Aspas A, Smith-Ballester S, García-Vigara A, Monllor-Tormos A, Kadi F, Nilsson A, Cano A. Nuts and metabolic syndrome: Reducing the burden of metabolic syndrome in Menopause. *Nutrients*. 2022;14:1677. https://doi.org/10.3390/nu14081677.

153. Silbiger JJ. Pathophysiology and echocardiographic diagnosis of left ventricular diastolic dysfunction. *J. Am. Soc. Echocardiogr.* 2019;32(2):216–232.e2.

Index

Note: Page numbers in *italics* indicate figures and in **bold** indicate tables on the corresponding pages.